Living with Type 1 D

Dr Tom Smith has been writing full time since 1977, after spending six years in general practice and seven years in medical research. He writes the 'Doctor, Doctor' column in the *Guardian* on Saturdays, and also has columns in the *Bradford Telegraph & Argus*, the *Lancashire Telegraph*, the *Carrick Gazette* and the *Galloway Gazette*. He has written three humorous books, *Doctor, Have You Got a Minute?*, *A Seaside Practice* and *Going Loco*, all published by Short Books. His other books for Sheldon Press include *Heart Attacks: Prevent and Survive*, *Living with Alzheimer's Disease*, *Coping Successfully with Prostate Cancer*, *Overcoming Back Pain*, *Coping with Bowel Cancer*, *Coping with Heartburn and Reflux*, *Coping with Age-related Memory Loss*, *Skin Cancer: Prevent and Survive*, *How to Get the Best from Your Doctor*, *Coping with Kidney Disease* and *Osteoporosis: Prevent and Treat*.

Overcoming Common Problems Series

Selected titles

A full list of titles is available from Sheldon Press,
36 Causton Street, London SW1P 4ST, and on our website at
www.sheldonpress.co.uk

Overcoming Common Problems Series

Overcoming Common Problems Series

Overcoming Common Problems

Living with Type 1 Diabetes

DR TOM SMITH

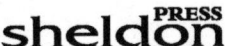
sheldon**PRESS**

First published in Great Britain in 2009

Sheldon Press
36 Causton Street
London SW1P 4ST

British Library Cataloguing-in-Publication Data
A catalogue record for this book is available from the British Library

ISBN 978–1–84709–052–2

1 3 5 7 9 10 8 6 4 2

Typeset by Fakenham Photosetting Ltd, Fakenham, Norfolk
Printed in Great Britain by Ashford Colour Press

Produced on paper from sustainable forests

Contents

Introduction

The greatest Olympian of all time and all countries is Britain's oarsman, Sir Steve Redgrave. He is the first athlete in endurance events ever to win gold in five successive Olympics, from 1984 to 2000.

He has type 1 diabetes.

If there was ever a role model for people with diabetes, insulin-dependent or otherwise, Sir Steve Redgrave is it. Of course, few people with diabetes can aspire to his athletic heights. But every one of them can take heart from the way he has put his body through the most rigorous training of all, yet still kept good control over his diabetes and remained super-fit.

Rowing is a punishing and gruelling sport. It is a huge feat to keep at the top for more than 16 years, even without diabetes. Without our current knowledge of diabetes, that task would surely have been insurmountable for someone with diabetes. How things have changed!

That's because we know so much more than we used to about how to control diabetes, and how to keep people with it free from harm, both in the short and long term. Sir Steve has obviously controlled his diabetes to perfection. The main aim of this book is to help others to emulate him – not in a search for Olympic gold, but at least to achieve the quality of life he so obviously enjoys, despite the health 'hiccup' of the discovery of his diabetes.

Because a health hiccup is what most people with diabetes have. Kept under good control, it cannot be looked upon truly as an illness in the sense that an illness could be defined as a state in which there are symptoms that make people feel unwell, and which can shorten life. In well-controlled diabetes, in which your glucose metabolism and all its ramifications have been returned to normal, you can feel as well, and live as long, as any person without diabetes. That isn't a description of an illness.

Although this book's aim isn't to make Olympians out of people with diabetes, it could help you to do just that, because the rules for diabetes affect everyone who has it, whether it started in childhood or in middle age, whether insulin is needed or not, and whether they are athletes or just average, everyday people. This book sets out the rules and describes the problems and pitfalls for people with diabetes, their families and carers, and how these problems can be faced and the pitfalls avoided.

When told for the first time that you have diabetes, you may have felt that you face a life sentence of poor health and an eventual early death. In the past it would have been a very unhappy time for children and their parents, as it would have been for you, as an adult who, perhaps, until the diagnosis would have been sailing on through life, unaware of the time bomb of troubles waiting to blow up in your face.

If you are going through this experience, then you can do what Sir Steve did: you can take a deep breath, put aside your fears, and look forward to a good and long life, just as enjoyable as everyone else's.

That doesn't mean, however, that you can live just like anyone without diabetes. You can't. You must stick closely to the correct healthy eating habits, take the correct amount of exercise, and comply with your medical team's advice on treatment, be it on insulin or glucose-lowering pills, or high blood pressure-lowering drugs. It is harder to be a child, teenager or adult with diabetes than one without it, but facing the challenge is worth the effort.

You have no alternative. If you don't face your particular challenge you may develop severe health problems. Teenagers who rebel against their fairly strict routine (unhappily a very common occurrence) are courting early blindness, kidney failure, heart attacks, strokes and circulation problems in their limbs. Adults with later-onset type 1 or type 2 diabetes can expect the same problems a few decades later if they don't manage to control their weight, their smoking habits and their blood pressure.

On the other hand, good control of diabetes and blood pressure in both children and adults, along with a healthy lifestyle, can greatly extend their length and quality of life, usually well into old age.

So this book describes all aspects of the healthy lifestyle that every diabetic needs to follow. It is positive and optimistic: it is more about 'dos' than 'don'ts'. It is full of hopes for the future: one chapter, for example, deals with the possibility of cure using modern transplant technology. Its main theme, however, is that you, and not your diabetes, will be in control of your own future.

Any book on type 1 diabetes should at least mention type 2. As we have learned more about the two conditions, we have realized that they have more in common than we used to think. So I have added a short chapter on type 2 diabetes, mainly for your information and interest, but partly also because the modern approaches to the two diseases are now very similar. I expect the main readership of the book, however, to be people with type 1 diabetes and their families.

1

Understanding diabetes

The full title of your disease is diabetes mellitus. 'Diabetes' is ancient Greek for 'siphon', or a constant flow of water, and 'mellitus' is from the Latin word for 'honey'. The two words describe the two main symptoms of the illness. Siphon refers to the constant need to drink water and pass urine, both in excess. Honey refers to the sweet, honey-like, taste of the urine, which is full of sugar, or to be more accurate, glucose. How did the older doctors know this? In the past, they made the diagnosis by tasting their patients' urine. Happily, as a twenty-first-century doctor, I do not have to do the same.

Diabetes mellitus is in fact two different diseases. One type usually starts in childhood, is caused by failure of the pancreas to produce insulin, and needs daily insulin injections. It is known by doctors as type 1 diabetes, childhood-onset diabetes and insulin-dependent diabetes mellitus (or IDDM). The other type, which usually starts in adulthood, is caused by the build-up in the body's tissues and organs of resistance to the action of insulin. This is type 2 diabetes, adult-onset diabetes and non-insulin-dependent diabetes (or NIDDM). People with it are still able to produce insulin, and can be treated largely by diet and if necessary by oral drugs.

However, in both types of diabetes, the general advice on lifestyle is similar, and the long-term complications are roughly the same, with both kinds of diabetes leading to higher risks of strokes and heart attacks, circulation problems, kidney failure and blindness. So, although this book is specifically aimed at adults with type 1 diabetes, much of it is relevant to people with type 2 diabetes and to teenagers with either type of diabetes.

What is it that makes it essential for people with diabetes to follow such a strict lifestyle? To answer this question we must understand some basic facts about the way our bodies process the sugars and starches in our food, which are the basis for all our energy needs.

The first essential is to understand the importance of glucose in the body. Glucose is the fuel that every cell in our body uses for its energy. We get it from the digestion of starches (mainly from bread, pasta, potatoes and rice) and sugars (mainly from fruit and sweets) in our food. All starches and sugars must be converted in our small intestine to glucose, which we can take up in the bloodstream so that it circulates around the body. Every cell in the body, no matter where or whatever its function, uses glucose as its basis for energy, and therefore for life. Without it the cell dies.

When we eat meals or drink liquids that contain starches and sugars, glucose levels start to rise in our blood – within a few minutes in the case of sugary drinks and after a longer time in the case of starches. Commonly this is described as a 'rising blood glucose'. The glucose has then to be transferred across the walls of the smallest blood vessels (the capillaries) into the tissues. With this transfer, the blood glucose starts to fall until we next swallow food or drink.

Once in the cells, the glucose is 'burnt' by oxygen to release energy that the cells can then use for all their functions, including the important one of staying alive. Oxygen arrives in the cells via the red blood cells, which pick it up in the lungs (from the air we breathe) and carry it through the heart and around the body to the capillaries. There the red cells give up the oxygen to be transferred through the capillary walls into the tissues, where it can reach the cells.

The whole process of burning glucose with oxygen could be compared with the internal combustion engine. In the cylinder of the engine, a spark of oxygen from the air intake causes a droplet of petrol to explode, providing the energy for the engine to run. In our human machine, we use the same oxygen, but this time the fuel is glucose. Like petrol, it is 'burnt', releasing energy for the cells to use, and finishing up as carbon dioxide and water, which we excrete through our lungs and kidneys, much like the exhaust pipes in a car.

How does this relate to diabetes? Glucose cannot reach the tissues on its own. We need insulin in the bloodstream to 'drive' the glucose from the blood across the capillary walls into the tissues. So shortly after eating or drinking sugary or starchy foods, not only does the blood glucose rise, but blood insulin levels rise, too. The pancreas, the organ that makes insulin, detects and responds to rising blood glucose levels by injecting insulin into the blood. As the blood insulin level rises, it drives the excess glucose into the tissues, where most of it is used to provide energy for the cells to perform their functions. Such functions could be the contraction of a muscle, a thought in the brain, the reception of light in the eye, a chemical process in the liver, or the filtering of waste from the blood by a kidney cell. All of these functions need glucose and oxygen, and all need insulin to get the glucose to the crucial spot.

One of our design faults as human beings is that we cannot store glucose in our cells. So for our bodies to keep active we need a constant supply of fresh glucose to our muscles, brain, heart, and all our other organs. We therefore must keep our blood glucose at the correct level, so that we never run short of our fuel. A car stops when the petrol flow to the cylinder fails. The same applies to a failure of glucose delivery to our cells: we shut down. Too low a blood glucose level, and we become 'hypoglycaemic' ('hypo' means 'under'; 'glyc' relates to 'glucose'; 'aemic' relates to 'haem' or 'blood'). A hypoglycaemic brain (a brain through which the flowing blood contains too little glucose) shuts down its activity to conserve energy, and we lose consciousness.

But too high a blood glucose level – which may occur when the mechanism that transfers glucose out of the capillaries into the tissues (i.e. insulin) has failed – may have the same result.

This is where diabetes comes in. Without enough insulin (as in type 1 diabetes) or when the insulin mechanism fails to shift the glucose out of the blood into the tissues (as in type 2 diabetes), blood glucose levels rise, because glucose cannot reach the cells. That, too, can lead to unconsciousness.

In essence, therefore, diabetes is simple to understand. We depend on a constant delivery of glucose to all our tissues for them to act normally and for us to survive. Insulin is the mechanism for doing precisely this – it could be compared with the fuel pump in a car. When the fuel pump goes wrong, no matter how much petrol we have in the tank, it can't reach the cylinder and the vital spark. Without a normal insulin mechanism, the glucose in our bloodstream can't reach the cells.

To complete the picture, we must add a little about the muscles and the liver. Glucose can be stored in both of these organs, but not as glucose itself. For storage, it must be converted into a more complex sugar, glycogen. Then, when we start to call on our immediate energy reserves – say when we are running or starving – we convert the glycogen back into glucose.

Muscles working at their limit convert stored glycogen into glucose and use it immediately. We surely have all experienced 'stitch': this is the pain we get when we have used up all the glycogen in our muscles and we start to run on 'empty'. The muscle uses fats instead, and that causes build-up of lactic acid inside them. The acid causes the typical pain of stitch. More than that, when fats are used instead of glucose for energy purposes, they do not break down, as glucose does, into carbon dioxide and water, but into 'ketones'. They are released in the urine, and sometimes in the breath. We shall have much more to say about ketones later.

The liver's glycogen stores are also a backstop against starvation and excessive exercise. Once the circulating glucose in the blood starts to fall below a critical level, the liver, like the muscles, converts stored glycogen into glucose and pushes it out into the bloodstream, from which the tissues can suck it out and use it.

So the normal person has two ways of providing glucose for the cells. One is directly via the glucose in the bloodstream that has appeared from the digestion of the last food and drink. The second is from the glycogen stores in the liver and the muscles.

The crucial thing to understand about both these processes is that they are wholly dependent on a normal insulin system. It is insulin that stimulates the release by the liver of glucose from its glycogen stores, and it is insulin that stimulates the conversion of glycogen into glucose inside the muscles.

So people with diabetes of either type have two major problems. They not only cannot get their circulating glucose into their cells, but they also cannot convert their glycogen stores into much needed glucose at times of high energy need.

Just think of coping with these two problems when you are an Olympic athlete, pushing your muscles to the normal limit and beyond, and marvel at Sir Steve's accomplishment! If he can get his insulin dose right to control his supply of glucose to his muscles and to manage his glycogen stores both to perfection, how much simpler it must be for you, with more ordinary problems, to manage yours!

2

Some case histories

It's easier to understand diabetes when you read about actual cases. If you have diabetes yourself, or are reading this to know more about a relative's diabetes, then you will surely recognize one of the following descriptions.

Chris
Chris was nine years old when he fell ill. Previously a completely normal little boy, doing well at school, the change in his health was dramatic. He was suddenly always thirsty, needing to drink far more often – and far more – than his brothers and sisters and his classmates. He was also visiting the toilet far more, to pass urine – a fact that his teacher noticed (because it disturbed his class) before his mother did (because he was quietly slipping off on his own at home to do it). He retained his healthy appetite, yet he was losing weight. From being a well-rounded little boy, he became noticeably thinner over only a week or two.

But most of all, he did not feel well. He had vague muscle pains, had a constant ache in his back, especially before passing urine, and he felt weak and tired. He could no longer keep up with his classmates in the school playground – from being a leader in games he became a watcher. His school work was suffering, too, in that he was sleepier than usual during the day and could not concentrate.

His teacher brought her worries about him to his mother, whose fears that he was ill were then confirmed. A rapid visit to the doctor led to a fast diagnosis and admission to the local children's ward for initial control of his type 1 diabetes and the start of his long-term self-management.

Now aged 45, Chris remembers the day he started on insulin as if it were yesterday. In his student years he played soccer for his university. He passed through the rigorous training as a medical student with relative ease and without any health problems. A doctor now, he keeps his diabetes under tight control, and has reaped the benefit of doing so, with a happy and healthy family life, and, so far, no complications. He helps hundreds of other people with diabetes in his large hospital diabetes clinic. He is a great example for them to follow.

Jane

In complete contrast to Chris's case, Jane didn't notice anything wrong until she was in her mid-40s. Even then, she assumed that her troubles were due to her approaching middle age and menopause. Her main worry was that she had lost weight – about 13kg (2 stone) in the previous few months. As she hadn't been much overweight before she had started to feel 'off' (her word for how she was feeling!) and hadn't been dieting, this had begun to worry her. She also felt less 'energetic', tending to drop off to sleep in the early evenings, and not feeling much like going out and doing things. She admitted to being 'a bit thirsty', and, for the first time in her life, to the need to get up once or twice every night to pass urine.

More embarrassingly, she complained of an itch around the vagina, and a discharge. This, too, was a first time for her. It had been a source of worry for her and her husband, who also had an itch. Happily, as a well-balanced couple, neither blamed the other for the problem.

Her doctor found large amounts of glucose in her urine, and confirmed her diabetes by performing a blood glucose test on the spot. She gently explained that Jane probably had type 2 diabetes and, after a few reassuring words, arranged for her and her husband to come back later that day. At that meeting she gave them the time they needed to learn much more about the illness and how they could cope with it. She and her husband were also given immediate treatment for her thrush infection, a common cause of genital itch in newly diagnosed or difficult-to-control diabetes.

Her doctor then introduced Jane to the rest of the practice diabetes team. In modern medical practice, most people with diabetes are 'managed' by the primary care team of general practitioner, specialized diabetic nurse and dietician. They had unexpected news for her. She was a puzzle, they said. Most people who develop diabetes in their 40s have the type 2 form of the illness. They are usually overweight, rather than underweight, and Jane's weight loss raised the suspicion that she had the type 1 form. Rather than simply arranging for her to go straight on to the usual regimen for type 2 diabetes, which would involve pills to improve her glucose control and advice on her eating habits and exercise, she was referred urgently to the local hospital diabetes clinic for further tests.

Once their results were through, Jane was started on insulin and was placed on the type 1 diabetes register. She took the news very well, settled in to her new lifestyle, and felt better almost immediately. Now, three years later, she sees her diagnosis of type 1 diabetes as a small 'blip' in her life that has made little difference to its quality. In fact, she told me only a few weeks ago that it was the stimulus to a new and far more satisfying relationship with her husband.

Before the diagnosis, she admitted, they had both been working full time in quite separate jobs, returning home at night often too tired to enjoy each other. The diagnosis had made them stop and think about health and mortality, perhaps for the first time in their busy lives. Once her diabetes had been stabilized they had taken a holiday together, she had changed her job to fit in better with his, and they now spent much more time together. Every aspect of their marriage, including their sex life, had improved immeasurably.

William

William prided himself on his fitness. He had been a long-distance runner at school, and he had continued the sport through teacher training college and into his job as PE teacher in a large comprehensive school. He was physically active at work and in his leisure time, completing several marathons each year and reaching county standard with times around two and a half hours. He ate healthily and was, he thought, perfectly healthy. At age 35 he was sailing through life with not a care in the world. He had a wife and two children, and they all enjoyed being physically active. They were the modern healthy family, slim and good-looking.

Except that William found that he was thirstier than he used to be. His appetite had 'improved', in that he was perpetually hungry: he was eating more than he used to, but was still not putting on weight – in fact he was losing weight. On his training runs, he felt that he became fatigued more easily than in the past, and he took a lot longer to recover from them than before. He put all these changes down to normal ageing, and didn't bother his doctor.

He should have: the combination of loss of weight with increased appetite in a previously normal person is a 'red flag' for one of two diseases – increased thyroid activity (we call it thyrotoxicosis) and diabetes. What brought him to his doctor's attention was the fact that one morning, not long after he started to feel this way, his wife, Eve, couldn't wake him up in the morning. She also noticed a strange sweet smell in the bedroom. She called her doctor, who alerted the emergency ambulance, and both arrived at the house at the same time. Luckily William had told Eve about how he was feeling, so the doctor had a head start with the diagnosis. The smell of acetone and a rapid finger-prick blood test showing a blood glucose level in the high 20s confirmed a diabetic coma, and an insulin injection started his treatment before he reached hospital.

William had adult-onset type 1 diabetes, and fortunately he quickly recovered from his initial 'event'. He wondered whether his excessively energetic lifestyle had 'brought on' his illness, but his diabetes specialist reassured him. In fact his fitness helped him to recover faster than would have been normally the case, and he was told that his diabetes was inevitable, regardless of the exercise he was doing.

William, like Sir Steve, is now a model patient, which isn't surprising considering his devotion to physical fitness before the illness appeared. He devotes as much of his attention to proper control of his diabetes as he did to his PE and his running. He is now 50 and still fit and well. So far he has had no complications, which is good considering that the episode that first brought him to his doctor's attention was a full-blown diabetic coma.

Anna

Anna and her husband married in their late 20s, but decided to put off having a family for a few years until they felt they could afford to give their children a good start in life. It's all too common a decision taken by twenty-first-century couples, and it's sometimes not for the best, health-wise.

They were delighted when, at 35, Anna eventually became pregnant. They had only been 'trying' for a few months, and they had both enjoyed excellent health until then. They foresaw no problems on their horizon. So Anna was very upset when, at her second antenatal visit, 12 weeks into her pregnancy, her routine urine sample showed a moderate amount of glucose. She had been feeling well, and so the news shocked her. Knowing a little about diabetes because an aunt had had it, she was fearful that her baby might be affected, and that she might fall ill during the pregnancy.

The antenatal team was able to reassure her. A 'fasting blood glucose level' was taken the next morning. This was a glucose measurement from blood taken before breakfast the morning after a light meal 12 hours before. It showed a glucose level a little higher than normal, a sign that she did have diabetes, but not necessarily one that would last beyond her pregnancy.

The next step was for her to have an 'oral glucose tolerance test' or OGTT. For this she was asked to swallow 50g of glucose, and blood glucose levels were measured just before doing so, then at regular intervals for a few hours afterwards. The OGTT showed that her blood glucose rose higher than normal and stayed there, only returning towards the normal level very slowly.

Anna was then sent to a diabetes team specializing in diabetes of pregnancy – gestational diabetes – where she was given advice on an anti-diabetic diet and on how to lose weight: she was more than 13kg (2 stone) overweight. She was taught how to measure her own blood glucose, and was not given anti-diabetic drugs.

For the rest of her pregnancy she was watched for any rise in glucose levels. Unfortunately, she found the diet difficult to follow, and although she didn't put on any more weight, her blood glucose level remained above the crucial levels of 6 millimoles per litre (mmol/l) before meals and 9mmol/l after meals. (There is more in later chapters on these measurements.) She had to be started on insulin.

Anna's pregnancy continued to full term, when she had a healthy baby boy weighing just over 3.6kg (8lb). The diabetes team gradually weaned her off the insulin. Thankfully, she stuck more closely to her diabetes team's advice on eating habits and the need for weight loss, so that by the six-week post-natal visit to her doctor, her blood glucose level was back to normal. However, she is not necessarily cured of her diabetes. About 40 per cent of women like Anna with gestational diabetes go on in later life to develop overt type 2 diabetes. She was warned of this fact, and has been asked to keep up her new lifestyle indefinitely.

She has been healthy now for ten years. She wears a size 12, she runs, walks, cycles and swims with her ten-year-old son and her admiring husband, and has every chance of avoiding diabetes if she continues as she has done.

Arthur

Arthur's story is not so hopeful. A heavy drinker since his teens, at 45 he started to feel decidedly unwell. His hangovers were lasting for longer than just the next morning. He felt sick most of the next day, and tended to take the 'hair of the dog' in the early evening to feel better. It didn't work.

What eventually brought him to his doctor was a constant pain right across the small of his back. It was so bad that he used a hot water bottle on the back to ease the pain, and in doing so burnt himself, leaving the skin red and blistered. By this time he had lost a lot of weight, and his appetite, too. He did not directly complain of thirst, but as he was in the habit of consuming large quantities of beer most days, a change in his fluid consumption and urine output might have been difficult to spot.

What his doctor did not find difficult to spot was that he looked ill and faintly jaundiced. His stomach was slightly swollen, and he was very tender when the doctor pressed his hand on his abdomen, just below the bottom of his breastbone.

Blood tests showed that Arthur had chronic pancreatitis, a condition very common in heavy drinkers. He needed to be taken off all alcohol, and he was admitted to hospital to try to reverse the damage and to see if the liver, too, was affected. During the extensive hospital tests he was found to have diabetes. Unlike the others described above, his diabetes was a direct result of the damage that alcohol had caused to his pancreas, which could no longer make enough insulin for his needs. In effect, he had a form of type 1 diabetes, even though it started when he was an adult.

Arthur's doctors told him that alcohol was now a virtual poison for him, and that his only hope of future health was to become teetotal, and to follow the strict insulin, diet and exercise rules that all people with type 1 diabetes must follow. He did that for several years, but eventually he failed to come to his regular follow-up appointments, and recently we heard through the grapevine that he had started drinking again. If this is true his health will deteriorate very quickly.

Sanji

Sanji was 43 when he attended a doctor for a routine medical assessment for life assurance, organized by his employer. He was astonished when he was refused insurance and was asked to see his own doctor for a check-up. Because life assurance doctors act for the insurers, and not for the 'insuree', he was not given any details about why he had been refused.

His own doctor, who had not seen him for years, picked up two solid reasons for his refusal. One was high blood pressure, the other was glucose in his urine ('glycosuria'). Sanji's first reaction to these test results was disbelief. Why, if he was so ill, he asked, did he not feel unwell? His doctor went over the last few years of Sanji's life in detail. Was he still doing the things he was doing five years ago, for example? Well, no, was the reply. He was no longer taking so much exercise. He had been promoted into a much more responsible job. It meant business dinners, late nights, many stressful decisions to make, and more time at his desk, in the car and on planes. He had put on about 13kg (2 stone) in weight, mostly around his middle. No, he had not noticed if he was less fit than before, but that was mainly because he could not remember when he last had enough physical exercise to make him breathless.

It turned out, when he had a fitness check on a treadmill, with a cardiac monitor strapped to his chest, that he was decidedly less fit than he thought. Not only was his OGTT verging towards diabetes, he had a high blood cholesterol level and high insulin levels, too.

His doctor diagnosed syndrome X, a combination of high blood pressure, high cholesterol, high blood glucose and central obesity (meaning that he was apple-shaped, with his main fat around his stomach, rather than pear-shaped, with the main fat around his buttocks and hips). This combination of problems is very well known to doctors, especially in people, like Sanji, whose parents originated from the Indian subcontinent, and is entirely due to the insulin resistance mentioned in the previous chapter. It needs very strict treatment to avoid an early death due to heart attack or stroke. And this is why Sanji had been refused his life assurance.

Give Sanji credit. Once his position had been made clear to him, he made some very important decisions about his life. He made sure he took time off to 'smell the roses'. More quality time with his family, more exercise, far better eating habits and learning to relax has made all the difference. Over the past five years, he has lost the extra weight, his blood pressure has fallen to normal levels and there is no glucose in his urine. However, his blood glucose levels, including his OGTT, did not return to within normal limits. His doctor gave him the usual pills to correct type 2 diabetes, but even they didn't correct the glucose control. He was started on small doses of insulin: as Sanji himself said, 'It worked like magic.'

He felt much better within a few days of starting insulin. His cholesterol level was more difficult to control, but it has eventually fallen after he started on a statin drug – about which more later. After all this time, a life assurance company has given him a policy that recognizes that he now has a future. But this is no cure. His syndrome X is under control, and will come back if he returns to his former habits. He is determined not to do so. How should his diabetes be defined? Officially it is classified as type 2, but the need for insulin to control it casts doubt on where the difference between the two types of diabetes lies. My feeling is that as he needs insulin, with all that this means for his future management, he should be considered as having type 1 diabetes. It's a moot point.

Eric

Eric was perfectly healthy until his 40th birthday. In a sedentary job (he is an accountant), he went to the local gym twice a week to 'keep himself fit'. Perhaps it was because of this that he ate very well: his favourite meal was fish or steak and chips. He smoked, too, 'only ten a day' he said, as if that wasn't serious enough to harm him. His only health problem was a high cholesterol level, found on a routine blood test, for which he refused to take a statin drug, because he felt that 'he was too thin for a heart attack', and he didn't want to take such a drug long term. He could wait for a few years, he told his doctor, before he 'had to self-medicate'.

He was wrong about that. His 40th birthday party was a grand affair, with all his family and friends around him. After plenty of rich food, good wine, a cigar or two, he went to bed, and slept like a stone – until four in the morning, when he woke up with an excruciating pain in his upper abdomen. At first he thought it was indigestion, but his usual over-the-counter indigestion tablets didn't help. His wife, seeing him in distress, phoned for an ambulance.

Over the next few days, he became very ill, with deepening jaundice. He was in intensive care for several days, before the pain eventually settled. Tests in that initial period showed that he had acute pancreatitis, so severely that his pancreas had 'necrosed'. It took months for him to recover, and he was left with insulin-dependent diabetes (because he was no longer able to make his own insulin) and a severe digestive disorder (because he could no longer produce the normal range of pancreatic enzymes needed to digest proteins in his food).

For the rest of his life Eric had to self-inject insulin, in exactly the same way as any person with type 1 diabetes, and to swallow the correct mix of pancreatic enzymes to allow him to digest his food. Luckily his wife was wonderfully supportive, and he has remained in reasonably good health for the next 30 years – a huge tribute to both of them. Today he self-injects four times a day. He still exercises several times a week, but he doesn't smoke, and he takes a statin drug to lower his cholesterol.

Why did he develop such a devastating pancreatitis? It was probably a combination of the high cholesterol with his smoking habit. The high fat levels in his blood led to the formation of gallstones, one of which may have slid down the 'common bile duct' to block its opening into the small bowel. In some people the pancreatic duct carrying the digestive enzymes into the bowel shares that opening. Blocking the one duct also blocked the other – and the back-flow of digestive juices started to digest his pancreas. The nicotine, tars and carbon monoxide in the smoke had damaged the fine blood vessels in his pancreas, making pancreatitis more likely and lowering the chances of recovery from it. It was a hard lesson for him – but he learned it.

Iain

Then there's Iain, the family doctor (no relation to Chris – it is just coincidence that two of my examples happen to be doctors). When he was 29, in rural general practice, he caught mumps. It surprised him because he had looked after many children with this infection of the glands in the cheeks without any thought that he might not have had it himself as a child. Obviously he hadn't. He woke one morning with what appeared to be a rugby ball broadside in his throat, and made his own diagnosis with a brief look in the mirror.

He was relatively lucky, in that he didn't develop the one complication that most men dread, orchitis (inflammation of the testes). But he did have a niggling pain in the centre of the upper abdomen, just under the ribs, that lasted the same time as the swollen glands in his neck. It wasn't a bad pain, and didn't stop him seeing patients who had had mumps. (Of course, he couldn't see patients who had not had mumps, in case he infected them.)

Four years later, Iain wasn't feeling too well. At 33 Iain had changed his job. Now in a research post, he spent far more time sitting, much less time walking and almost no time in vigorous exercise. He had slowly gained about 13kg (2 stone), almost without noticing. He was sleepy in the evenings, hadn't his usual energy even to mow the lawn and was getting a bit short-tempered with his long-suffering wife and two small children.

It was his wife, who has no medical or nursing training, who suggested he might be diabetic. He laughed at the preposterous suggestion, but took a urine sample, just the same. It contained glucose. He says it's a good, even humbling, lesson for any doctor. Iain firmly believes that every doctor should have a similar experience, to learn what it is like at the wrong end of the stethoscope.

He was lucky. He had to lose the weight, start exercising again and eat healthily, and his OGTT, which had been in the diabetic range, returned to normal. His specialist thought that the abdominal pain he had with the mumps was a mild pancreatitis. The virus had inflamed his pancreas, as well as his salivary glands. This had reduced his capacity to produce insulin. In effect he was on the way to a type 1 diabetes if he continued to pursue such a sedentary lifestyle. On the other hand, if he doesn't put too much load on what remains of his pancreas, it will produce enough insulin for all normal needs. It is a rare cause of diabetes, but one to be taken into account in anyone who has had pancreatitis in the past.

From the day of Iain's diagnosis he changed his tastes. He took no more sugar in tea and coffee, and no more sugar-filled desserts. His source of carbohydrates from then on was bread, pasta, rice and potatoes, plus fresh fruit. He never ate more than he needed, and often rose from the table still feeling a little hungry. Even now, many years later, he feels hungry most of the time. A little exercise every day, he says, takes the edge off this excessive appetite.

When he was given the diagnosis, Iain started running again, and felt better within a few days. He has kept it up over the years, and now runs half-marathons with his teenage sons. He doesn't aim for the times that William, for example, still achieves: he runs for fun and general fitness, and not competitively, so a half-marathon in just over two hours is good enough for him. His boys finish 30 minutes ahead of him, but he doesn't mind. He gave up his research job, and went back to practice, using his experience to run the diabetes clinic. His own OGTT is normal, he no longer has glucose in his urine and his fasting blood glucose is around 3–4mmol/l. At six feet tall, he does not let his weight rise above 80kg (13 stone).

These case histories were chosen because of their diversity, and yet they have a common strain running through them – the fact that for everyone with diabetes of whatever cause or type, it isn't just a matter of taking glucose-lowering drugs or insulin. It is just as much a matter of lifestyle and obeying the healthy living rules. You may have found your own history, or something close to it, among these case histories. The chapters that follow use these cases to illustrate how diabetes is managed and the problems and pitfalls that may affect people like them.

The aim in every case is not just to keep people relatively well. Probably the most apt statement on the treatment of diabetes is by Professor Robert Tattersall, a much respected British diabetic specialist and researcher. 'Diabetes', he wrote, 'is an easy disease to treat badly.' The aim of the next few chapters is to make sure that you treat yourself well, because you are the main person in your treatment. Others can only give advice. You are the only person who can put that advice into practice.

If your diabetes is badly treated, you may avoid the immediate problems of comas and 'hypos' – about which more later. But you will be laying yourself open to serious complications over the next 20 years or so – such as heart attacks, strokes, blindness, kidney failure and gangrene of the limbs. We know now that good blood glucose control and good blood pressure control – the two go hand in hand in diabetes – will greatly help to prevent them all. The next few chapters put these risks into context and spell out exactly why you should be strict with yourself, so that you can avoid them.

A final point about these histories, all of which are based on actual patients I have seen in my years of general practice, is that they show that the distinction between type 1 and type 2 diabetes is blurred. We used to call the two types of diabetes 'juvenile' diabetes and 'maturity-onset' diabetes, the first being dependent on insulin and the second being usually controlled by better lifestyle and possibly 'antidiabetic' pills. This classification was changed to type 1 diabetes (caused by loss of insulin production) and type 2 diabetes (caused by resistance to the action of insulin) about 20 years ago, in an attempt to base it on better knowledge of the mechanisms underlying the two forms of the disease, and to establish rational ways of treating it.

One of the reasons for the change was that, as people are becoming more obese earlier in life, every family doctor now has teenagers with what used to be called maturity-onset diabetes. It's a sad reflection on our changing times and the obesity pandemic. And we seem to be seeing more people who develop what was defined as 'juvenile' diabetes in adult life – Sir Steve and William are good examples. Even more complicated, we are now finding that a much higher proportion of our patients with so-called type 2 diabetes are needing insulin to control them. In effect they have type 2 diabetes, but they need classical type 1 treatment. That's why I've decided, in a book mainly on type 1 diabetes, to include sections on type 2. The treatment of both types of diabetes involves a lot of common ground, and for many of you, the two types of diabetes may well overlap. So please bear with me if some of the areas of the book are not entirely relevant to your case.

For the sake of completion on the subject of whether you have type 1 or type 2 diabetes, here are the official definitions in the *British National Formulary* – the guidebook on treatment of disease provided for British doctors by the British Medical Association and the Royal Pharmaceutical Society of Great Britain. In effect it is our 'Bible' on all matters medical.

> Type 1 diabetes (formerly referred to as insulin-dependent diabetes mellitus or IDDM) occurs as a result of a deficiency of insulin following autoimmune destruction of pancreatic beta cells. Patients with Type 1 diabetes require administration of insulin.
>
> Type 2 diabetes (formerly non-insulin-dependent diabetes mellitus or NIDDM) is due either to reduced secretion of insulin or to peripheral resistance to the action of insulin. Although patients may be controlled on diet alone, many also require oral antidiabetic drugs or insulin or both to maintain satisfactory control. In overweight individuals, type 2 diabetes may be prevented by losing weight and increasing physical activity.

It's clear from these definitions that the dividing line between the two, for practical purposes, is difficult to draw. So much of what follows is relevant to both types of the disease.

3

Tackling type 1 diabetes: the theory

Chris's diagnosis (see Chapter 2) was made more than 30 years ago, when he was nine years old. At that time, the main aim of managing diabetes in children was to control their diabetes so that they were reasonably able to live a normal life. The emphasis then was on three essentials – eating correctly, exercising and using their insulin injections in tune with their food intake, and their exercise.

Children around Chris's age with diabetes would be taught how to give their own insulin injections and how to recognize when things were getting out of control. They had to know themselves when they were 'hypo' or 'hyper', and how to treat either state. But as long as they kept in reasonably good glucose balance, their doctors felt satisfied that they were doing well.

Nowadays we know this is not nearly enough, either for children or adults with type 1 diabetes. Today's aim is not just to avoid the unpleasant symptoms of disturbed glucose levels, but also to try to keep the blood glucose pattern throughout the whole 24 hours as close to normal as possible. It is easy to keep the glucose levels within a broad band so that you feel relatively well and have no acute problems, but if we wish to do as much as we can to ward off the later complications, such as kidney failure, heart attacks, strokes and blindness, we need to do much more.

So today's type 1 diabetics must place much more emphasis than ever before on eating healthily, on regular exercise (particularly to keep the weight normal) and on the timing and doses of their insulin. They must also have regular checks on blood glucose levels, blood pressure, the eyes, the kidneys and the nervous system.

Luckily Chris's parents had had the foresight to make sure that he understood the importance of good diabetic control. This he knew at primary school. They also recognized that the danger time was in adolescence, and took special care to ensure that he passed through this turbulent phase as easily as possible. Chris was fortunate that, in wanting to become a doctor, he was particularly interested in the illness and its complications. His teenage years were spent mainly in studying and in trying to make the county's athletics team. His career choice and leisure preferences kept him on the straight and narrow, although he would admit now, looking back, that there were times when he could so easily have gone wrong.

Getting the control right in type 1 diabetes

The first priority in type 1 diabetes is to get the control right. This can only be done by co-ordinating as finely as possible three things – your intake of food, your physical activity and your dose and type of insulin. You must check yourself whether you are getting it right by regular blood glucose tests, and your doctor or diabetes nurse will double-check by performing a glycosylated haemoglobin (HbA1c) test.

HbA1c measurements

HbA1c is a measure of how well you have been controlling your blood glucose levels over the previous two to three months.

The principle of the HbA1c test is fairly easy to understand. With glucose floating about in the bloodstream all the time, some of it 'sticks' to the haemoglobin, the red pigment inside the red blood cells that carries oxygen around the body. This is known as glycosylated haemoglobin or HbA1c. Only around 4 per cent of the red cells are glycosylated in non-diabetics: this is read as an HbA1c of 4 per cent. The normal range is taken as between 3 per cent and 6.5 per cent.

In poorly controlled diabetes, in people whose blood glucose levels have been well above normal for many weeks on end, HbA1c can be above 20 per cent. Many people with reasonable control of their diabetes have HbA1c levels under 8 per cent.

That is important, because it has been proved time and again that lowering the HbA1c lowers the risk of later complications in the eyes, kidneys, nervous system and blood vessels. The risk of all of them rises substantially as the HbA1c climbs above 8 per cent.

Management of diabetes: an example from Denmark

Keeping the HbA1c low isn't simply a matter of getting the food, exercise and insulin about right. Particularly for children, it means receiving attention from several different professionals. Even in a sophisticated country like Denmark as recently as 1997, diabetic centres specializing in children were reporting average HbA1c levels of 9.4 per cent. The Danish specialists in childhood diabetes, shocked by their poor performance, therefore decided to reorganize the work of all the medical and paramedical staff to try to improve things. What follows is a model for the management of all type 1 diabetes, not just for children but for adults, too.

The first step was to establish a single centre for children's diabetes in Copenhagen. In October 2000 the staff were looking after 203 children. With around 33 new cases per year, by 2010 they will have more than 500 children in their care. Thirty per cent of them are under school age.

In starting their new approach to diabetes, the Copenhagen group had to admit that, despite technical improvements like better ways of measuring blood glucose at home, regular HbA1c tests, better ways of delivering the insulin (mainly with pens – see later), and more choice of insulins, they had not, in the previous ten years, improved the children's diabetes control. To do so, they reasoned, they must increase the children's self-confidence and self-sufficiency, so that they could better come to terms with their diabetes and how to control it. They had to involve and inform the whole family about diabetes, and improve the family's knowledge and skills. They had to attend to the special needs of ethnic minorities with language problems and of those with learning difficulties. They had to bring the family into the management plans and adapt these plans to the family's circumstances. They used the children's own experiences to help treat and provide support for newly diagnosed children.

It meant a lot of work and time, but it succeeded. All the children were treated as outpatients. Diabetic nurse specialists were employed, weekly meetings of the whole diabetic team were held to discuss problems in specific families coming to the clinic. Families had a 24-hour dedicated hotline to ring for problems. A children's psychologist was brought in, and the staff were given extra education in diabetes management.

The regular team now consists of specialist physicians in childhood diabetes, children's general physicians, specialist nurses, dieticians, chiropodists, laboratory technicians, social workers and psychologists.

Aims of the centre

They laid down the following aims for the children:

- to achieve normal growth and development;
- to achieve normal schooling and career goals;
- to achieve the optimum quality of life;
- to have understanding appropriate to their age about diabetes treatment;

- to keep as low as possible the complications of diabetes that can affect children (such as eye, kidney and nerve problems);
- to train the children to take over their own management at the appropriate age for them; and
- to transfer them to an adult clinic at the appropriate time.

The overall aim was to equip the children with all that they needed to care for their own diabetes for the rest of their lives.

Achieving those aims

The system involves great attention to detail. At the age of nine years every child has three very important examinations –their eyes, their kidneys and their nervous system. Their eyes are examined by a specialist ophthalmologist for the earliest evidence of 'diabetic retinopathy', the condition that in the past has led to blindness in so many type 1 diabetics.

They have two overnight samples of urine examined for microalbuminuria, tiny amounts of protein in the urine that predict later diabetic kidney disease. They have their nervous system examined for loss of the ability to detect vibration against the skin of the feet. That predicts later diabetic neuropathy (in which there is loss of sensation in the limbs) which can be the first stage in the pathway towards serious damage to the feet.

If the test results are normal and the HbA1c is under 8 per cent, then the child is screened again at age 11 and once a year thereafter. If they are not, then they are seen much more often, and every effort is made, with better control, to return them to normal.

How was the control improved? Parents and children were encouraged to measure blood glucose levels at home much more often than before, and to adjust the insulin dose, diet and physical activity according to the results. The diabetic nurses visit far more often than before – in the first six months at least twice a month, then every two to three months after establishing good control. The dietician, social worker and psychologist visit as required. Every child has a blood glucose meter and the results are read by a computer program that makes it much easier to adjust the treatment. Children of similar ages and their parents are encouraged to meet regularly to swap information and to be taught new and practical techniques. These sessions are very well attended!

Puberty – the problem years

Puberty is a problem for most people, whether or not they have diabetes. But it is particularly hard for children with diabetes. The rush of sex hormones, their changing energy needs (from excessive to slothful), their rapid growth, allied to psychological problems, makes good control very difficult. The diabetic teenager going out with non-diabetic friends to parties must still strictly control his or her behaviour in a way that seems unfair, and they can often resent it. Only too often they can let themselves go, and that, sadly, can lead to permanent damage to eyes, kidneys and nerves that will not repair.

So the teenager with diabetes must have a special counsellor who knows the problems, not just of diabetes but of teenagers, too. Such counsellors are pretty rare, but the Danes have concentrated on finding and training them. They communicate with adolescents on their own terms and negotiate realistic targets of control that their patients can accept. Teenagers with type 1 diabetes in Copenhagen attend after-school meetings arranged by the specialist nurses and dieticians. They discuss teenage diet, alcohol, how to cope with parties, contraception, worries about pregnancy and childbirth – in fact all the things that other teenagers need advice on, but rarely get.

Because continuity of care through the teenage years is so vital, teenage diabetics do not leave the children's diabetic system until they are 18 – three years after children's hospitals normally pass on their patients to adult clinics. Before the final transfer, there are three or more years of overlap, so that the adult team has got to know the new patient while he or she is still under the children's team care. That is vital, because it ensures continuity and builds trust in the new team. During the period of transfer, all the teenagers transferred at the same time meet informally together, consolidating that trust, and learning about the way the new medical team will continue to help them.

By the time they have reached the adult clinic, all the children who have gone through the Copenhagen scheme have become expert in their own care. They have gone through education schemes prepared jointly by the hospital, schoolteachers and psychologists. They possess information sheets and guidelines on coping with diabetes, and are tested on their knowledge of their diabetes, so that they can be re-trained if it is found wanting. Included in the education process are parents and grandparents, school friends, and teaching personnel in further education institutes.

Hitting the targets

Did the Danish team hit their targets? They were difficult ones to achieve. Where children had HbA1c levels of 10 per cent or above, they aimed to lower them to 9 per cent within a year. They aimed at HbA1c levels for the children aged under six to be below 9 per cent and for those aged seven to 18 years to be below 8.5 per cent in the first two years of diagnosis, and for all children to have HbA1c levels under 8 per cent within four years.

One reason for the higher (less strict) HbA1c target for the younger children was to avoid bringing the glucose level too low, and thereby causing the occasional severe hypoglycaemic attack, defined as a bout of unconsciousness and convulsions (fits). Such attacks in young children may cause brain damage, leading later to a lower intellect and to psychological problems. The clinic's aim was to keep their frequency to below 20 for every 100 patients treated for a year. They far exceeded this aim, with no 'hypos' in the younger children and only three in the older ones. Therefore, they reduced the average HbA1c even of the younger children to 8 per cent.

Another aim was to avoid repeated attacks of ketosis. 'Hypo' attacks are the result of the child receiving too much insulin for the amount of glucose circulating in the blood. This can happen when either the dose is too high or when not enough food is eaten after the injection. Ketosis is the opposite. If there is too little insulin in the circulation, the body must use fats, rather than glucose, for its energy source.

Unlike glucose, which breaks down into carbon dioxide and water when releasing its energy, fats break down into ketones, acid-like chemicals that appear in the breath and the urine, and for which there are simple urine tests. Ketones smell sweet, somewhat like pear drops, so they can be very obvious to people who can smell them (a substantial proportion of the population, including myself, can't). Ketosis is a sign that the person is on the way to a diabetic coma, and it should be corrected as soon as possible. That is best done by giving insulin and extra fluids.

The Danish team was highly successful in all their aims. The average HbA1c level in all their children fell from over 9 per cent to 8 per cent. The fall in the teenagers was even greater, from well over 10 per cent to around 7 per cent. Hypo attacks were almost eradicated in doing so – a considerable achievement, for the lower the HbA1c becomes, the greater the chance that on some days the blood glucose has dipped to low, and brought on a 'hypo'. None of the children had repeated ketotic attacks.

These Danish results are the best example of diabetes care I can find in the medical literature. The attention to education, care and follow-up are a model for every group involved in diabetes. If you feel that the care you or your children are receiving fall short of this standard, you should seriously consider why, and talk to your medical team about it. It is long past the time that diabetes was simply a matter of keeping free of 'hypos' and ketosis. That is the easy part. The difficult part is how to keep healthy and free of diabetes-related illness in your future. Before I go into how you can do that, however, there are practical points to consider about the day-to-day management of your insulin treatment and of the tests that ensure you are getting things right.

4

'Hypers', ketoacidosis and 'hypos'

When you are a newly diagnosed type 1 diabetic the first priority is to recognize how it feels to have hyperglycaemic attacks ('hypers') and hypoglycaemic ('hypo') attacks ('hypos') and to know precisely what to do when they start.

'Hypers'

Hyperglycaemia is uncontrolled diabetes – that is, your blood glucose is too high, mainly because you do not have enough circulating insulin to drive the glucose from the blood into the tissues, so that it cannot be used for all your energy purposes.

One problem with hyperglycaemia is that when the glucose is only moderately raised, you may notice nothing wrong at first. It is only when it persists and becomes much higher that you start to feel unwell. This is one reason why it is never enough just to sail along on the same dose of insulin day by day without checking blood glucose levels or HbA1c levels. You may have a constantly raised blood glucose, which can be quietly doing you damage without you knowing anything about it.

In fact if you have been 'hyper' for long periods you may not recognize how unwell you have been until your glucose levels are brought under stricter control. You then find out, perhaps for the first time in years, how it feels to be well. People with poorly controlled type 1 diabetes are often hyperglycaemic all the time, with spikes of even higher blood glucose levels after meals.

Once the 'hyper' symptoms start, though, you do become very aware of them. An early one is blurred vision, as the lens in the eye changes shape. High glucose levels are a fertile breeding ground for bacteria, while at the same time they interfere with your defences against infection. So you are much more prone to infections wherever a body surface meets the environment – like the skin and lungs. Recurring boils that do not heal and repeated chest infections can be the first hint of both type 1 and type 2 diabetes.

Rising blood glucose levels interfere with the brain, dulling the intellect and the ability to concentrate and making people lethargic and sleepy. The higher than normal blood glucose levels also overpower the kidney's ability to retain the glucose in the bloodstream, so it appears in the urine. The more glucose there is in the urine, the more water the kidneys have to excrete along with it, so hyperglycaemia brings with it excessive urine excretion. In short, you pass more urine more often than normal, day and night. The depletion of your body water makes you thirsty, so you drink more, too.

Urine is not a matter of water alone, however. It contains minerals, such as sodium, potassium and magnesium, essential to the workings of many organs, including the muscles. So as you pass more urine, you lose more minerals, too. Lacking essential minerals the muscles become less efficient, so you develop cramp and weakness on top of the tiredness and lethargy.

If this process continues for any length of time, because your body no longer has access to glucose as its source of energy (it is all trapped in the circulation and can't get to the tissues), it uses its stored fatty tissue instead. This produces loss of weight that can be quite drastic. In undiagnosed type 1 diabetes the weight loss can be 15kg (3½ stone) or more in a month or two. By then your urine is full of ketones as well as glucose.

Finally, if the diabetes is completely out of control, you become dehydrated, with glucose levels rising steeply, you become breathless and you lose consciousness, lapsing into coma.

It is to be hoped that no person with diagnosed type 1 diabetes should reach this final state. Long before it is reached, the initial symptoms of blurred vision, lethargy, poor concentration, thirst and excessive urine production, cramps and weakness, and the smell of ketones in the breath should have made the diagnosis obvious, and the correct treatment should have been started. But it is as well for all people with diabetes, and their family, to be very well acquainted with the possibility and to know exactly what to do when confronted with it.

Sometimes a hyper is easy to miss. For example, it could be mistaken for drunkenness, especially after people have had a drink or two and forgotten to take their insulin. Diabetics have also been known to forget to take their insulin with them on a journey, and decided to take the risk of missing a dose or two. Hyperglycaemia can creep up on them without them noticing, and they can quickly become too confused to tell people about it. Teenagers may deliberately do without their insulin dose as an act of rebellion against their disease and the discipline of managing it. They, too, can be mistakenly diagnosed as drunk at, say, a party, when the real cause is lack of insulin and consequent hyperglycaemia.

So it is incumbent on everyone with diabetes and their family to be as expert as their doctors in recognizing the signs of early hyperglycaemia and correcting it as soon as possible. That means people with type 1 diabetes must always make sure that they have their insulin delivery kit and preferably their blood glucose monitoring kit with them at all times. They should also wear a Medicalert disc so that anyone finding them in a semi-conscious state knows who they are and whom to contact for help.

Ketoacidosis

Ketosis (or ketoacidosis) is the end-result of neglected hyperglycaemia. All people with type 1 diabetes must always be aware of how it feels to become ketotic, because recognizing it and reversing it in time can save their lives. As explained in Chapter 1, when the body is unable to use glucose as a source of energy, it has to turn for energy directly to the fat stored in the fatty tissues. Even non-diabetic people who have not eaten for a day or so, and have therefore depleted their liver and muscle stores of glycogen (see p. 3), must start breaking down their body's fat stores. It is the mechanism we use when we are starving.

As explained earlier, using fat directly in this way (we normally convert it into glucose first, then use insulin to pump it into the organs and tissues) leads to ketones as a waste product. Ketones build up in the bloodstream, and the excess appears in the urine, in which it can be detected by simple 'strip' tests. Normal urine, passed by non-diabetics who are not starving or by diabetics under good control, does not contain any detectable ketone.

In poorly controlled or undiagnosed type 1 diabetes (with too little insulin activity, or too much carbohydrate intake, or both), rising blood ketone levels lead to trouble. This is because they are acid. The body's metabolism is organized so that it works most efficiently when all the body's fluids (in the blood and in the fluid in and around the tissues and organs, including the brain and muscles) are slightly alkaline. As the ketone levels build up, the body's ability to keep the acid–base balance precisely as it should be (for the technically minded, a pH level of around 7.3–7.4) fails, and the body becomes 'acidotic' (the pH drops, so that in extreme cases it can fall below 7.0).

In this state of ketoacidosis, none of the organs work well. The brain, liver and kidneys start to fail, so you become tired and sleepy, feel sick and indeed can be very sick. Because your kidneys excrete far more fluid than normal, you quickly become parched. Your mouth dries up, and you breathe very deeply (doctors call this Kussmaul breathing) and, if it is allowed to continue, you will become unconscious. This is a diabetic coma.

Before we had insulin, ketoacidosis and coma was the usual cause of death in diabetes. It takes about 24 hours to progress from the start of ketoacidosis to coma, so there should always be time to prevent it from becoming a serious threat to life, as long as the early signs are recognized and are properly treated.

How do you recognize if you are slipping into ketoacidosis? The initial change is becoming more thirsty and passing more urine than normal, particularly if your blood glucose level is over 17mmol/l. If at any time your blood glucose is at this height you must check your urine for ketones. If the result is positive, then check again in three to four hours. If ketones are still present, then you must contact your clinic urgently for advice, unless you have specific instructions designed just for you in these circumstances.

The number of cases of ketoacidosis are, thankfully, very rare among today's type 1 diabetics. This is partly because they are now under regular management. All diabetics in the UK should be under a general practice or hospital diabetes management team, and should therefore be well aware of the problem and how to avoid it. However, it won't do any harm in listing here the ways it can occur and how to avoid them.

Causes of ketoacidosis

The most common causes of ketoacidosis are still too much food or too little exercise. Problems arising from either can be prevented by keeping to regular eating and exercise patterns, and by increasing the insulin dose when increasing food or reducing exercise. You may have to use trial and error to find out how you should change the insulin dose, with the guidance of your diabetic specialist nurse or doctor. Each person is different, and it would not be useful here to describe dose schedules in detail, because what suits one person may well not suit another.

Developing ketoacidosis may be a gradual process because your insulin needs may change as time passes. One way of preventing its onset is to monitor your blood glucose levels carefully: if over days and weeks they are gradually rising, you may have to increase your insulin dose by between 2 and 8 units per injection. This, too, should be discussed with your diabetes nurse or doctor.

A single forgotten insulin dose isn't likely to produce ketoacidosis. And it can be put right according to simple rules. For example, if you are injecting insulin twice daily, and remember before midday that you have forgotten your morning dose, take between half and two-thirds of the dose immediately. If you don't remember it until the evening then check your blood glucose and get on your usual diabetes 'hotline' to discuss the appropriate dose with the nurse or doctor. Most people nowadays take four injections a day: forgetting one of them should not cause any serious problem and there is no need to adjust the next dose.

Probably the most difficult time for someone with type 1 diabetes is during another illness, particularly an infection, or when under physical or mental stress. This can also bring on ketoacidosis if not managed correctly. Being in an accident, undergoing an operation, having anxiety or depression, or even something as simple as a common cold or 'flu, can push up your blood glucose level. How much higher it gets varies widely from person to person, so again it isn't easy to give precise instructions here on how to raise the insulin dose to compensate.

In these circumstances the rule is to check your blood glucose level once every four hours or so while you are ill or under unusual stress. You may have to increase your insulin levels by between 4 units up to double your usual dose, depending on the height of your blood glucose levels. Experience will tell you how much extra you need, and as always be guided by your diabetes nurse or doctor.

A particular risk is posed by an illness that stops you eating, makes you vomit or gives you diarrhoea. Gastroenteritis, for example, may give you all three. It is vital not to stop your insulin: just because you cannot take in food does not mean that you must lower your insulin dose accordingly. This is a mistake often made by new diabetics when they develop such an illness for the first time after their diagnosis. Instead, you must measure your blood glucose level more often than usual, and increase your insulin accordingly if it is climbing. At the same time you should try to swallow fluids that contain carbohydrate.

Foods that are useful sources of fast glucose during illnesses include glucose itself, sugar, jams, marmalades and honey, undiluted fruit squashes and juices, lemonade, tinned milk puddings, drinking chocolate, and nutritional powders normally reserved for invalids.

If while you are ill, and particularly you are being sick and are getting dehydrated, your urine is positive for ketones, then you must immediately contact your usual diabetes expert contact (usually via a hotline). If it continues for more than four or five hours, then get someone to take you to the local hospital accident and emergency department.

If you are isolated, and cannot get into hospital, and you know your diabetes is getting much worse, with ketones and a rising blood glucose, then until you can reach medical help follow the following rules:

- inject 4 units of a fast-acting insulin (see Chapter 6) once an hour;
- check your blood glucose once an hour until it falls to normal for you; and
- drink at least 600ml (1 pint) of water every hour until you return to normal.

If you are a 'brittle' diabetic so that you have such problems fairly often and you live in an area where it is difficult to reach professional help easily, it is a good idea to place the above list in a prominent place where everyone in the house can see it. And they can all be taught how to give your injections, too, so that they can help even when you are too confused or sleepy to do it yourself.

'Hypos'

Hypoglycaemia is likely to happen when the blood glucose drops below 3mmol/l. In North America this is equivalent to 55 milligrams per decilitre (mg/dl). A hypo produces hunger, dizziness, sweating, trembling, slurred speech, faintness, confusion and palpitations (a fluttering feeling in the chest due to fast heartbeats). If not treated urgently, the person loses consciousness and may even convulse (have a fit).

All patients with type 1 diabetes must be able to recognize how they feel when becoming hypoglycaemic. Your pattern of symptoms is unique to you, and you must be able to recognize the symptoms early so that you can reverse the hypoglycaemia before you are unable to do so. Your doctors may even give you a deliberate 'hypo' so that you can recognize your symptoms, and know how to deal with it efficiently.

A particular type of 'hypo' is the type that happens when you are asleep. If you have spent a restless night with perhaps a nightmare, and wake with a headache, you probably have had a hypo in the small hours. Paradoxically, you may find that your blood glucose the following morning is higher than usual. This is despite urine tests taken at the same time being free of glucose, but positive for ketones. To prevent such night-time hypos you should have a bedtime snack.

Patterns of hypos may change over the years. In particular you may lose the first warning signs (usually sweating and trembling). You need to be alert to this change and to recognize the other signs. If you are less aware of your hypos, you may need to lower your insulin dose or change your insulin type. See later for more details about insulin use.

Causes of hypos

The main causes of hypoglycaemic attacks are delaying or missing meals after giving yourself an insulin dose. You should be very strict about regular mealtimes and about your regular snacks between meals and before sleeping. Other causes include an accidental overdose of insulin. If you realize that this has happened within a short time, you can usually prevent a serious hypo by taking extra glucose. If it is a high overdose (say twice your usual or more) then tell your doctor at once.

Unplanned extra physical activity can also induce hypo attacks, so every type 1 diabetic should carry a stock of glucose (such as Dextrosol tablets) or lump sugar in a pocket or handbag. Sometimes an action as simple as running for a bus or having to climb stairs when a lift is out of order may precipitate a hypo.

Finally, there is alcohol. Moderate to heavy drinking can interfere with the body's control of the balance between blood glucose and insulin, so that it can increase the risk of a hypo even when you have otherwise eaten normally and taken the right dose of insulin. People with type 1 diabetes should never binge drink, and should always eat whenever they are drinking.

Dealing with hypos

As repeated hypo attacks can harm the brain, they should be avoided as far as possible. The easiest way to do so is to carry on your person, all the time, a packet of glucose (dextrose) tablets. Even if the attack is a mild one, a tablet chewed at the first symptom can be essential to prevent it becoming more serious. A more severe attack can be quickly corrected by a drink of sweetened milk and a sweet biscuit. If you become too drowsy too quickly to deal with them yourself, the instructions on your Medicalert bracelet should be clear enough for people near you to feed you a sweet drink before you lose consciousness. You should make sure that your immediate friends and family all know how to recognize a hypo and how to deal with it.

Hypostop is a glucose-rich jelly in a tube that can be squeezed like toothpaste into the mouth of people in hypo attacks, and if necessary rubbed on to the gums. In an emergency, if the hypo is causing the person to lapse into unconsciousness, then a doctor will inject glucose solution into a vein. People who are prone to repeated hypo episodes may be prescribed injections of glucagon, a hormone that has the opposite effect to insulin. It comes in the form of ampoules in a kit, with which friends and family must make themselves familiar. It is given as a 1mg injection of 1ml of solution into the thick muscle just below the shoulder on the outside of the upper arm. People coming round after a glucagon injection often feel sick, but the feeling clears over an hour or so.

A point that cannot be made too strongly is that repeated hypo attacks should be avoided, because of the danger of long-term brain damage. In the past, when insulin injections were given only once or twice a day as a mixture of short-acting and long-acting preparations, people tended to tolerate the odd hypo as the price to pay for keeping the blood glucose levels as low as possible. This is no longer the case. Today's treatment involves several injections of different types of insulin throughout the day, planned to fit with small and frequent meals. Individual insulin doses are now lower than they were and, in a person with well-controlled type 1 diabetes, blood levels of both insulin and glucose do not fluctuate nearly as widely as was common only a few years ago.

With the much better control of both insulin and glucose levels, hypo attacks should be a thing of the past for most type 1 diabetics. If you are having them, and have been unable to control them yourself, then you must discuss it as a matter of high priority with your diabetic specialist.

Why insulin?

It would be great if insulin could just be swallowed, like other medicines for, say, arthritis, but it can't. Because it is a protein, our digestive juices in the stomach would simply break it down, so that we could not absorb it. For it to reach our tissues and bloodstream we must inject it. In the near future we may make much more use of insulin delivery by nasal spray, because the delicate lining membranes of the nose can absorb it. Nasal sprays would be marvellous if they were reliable – anyone would prefer using them to having injections – but their main snag is that insulin doses must be precise for good control, and the ability of our nasal membranes to absorb insulin varies hugely when we have allergies such as hay fever or colds. We don't yet know how to direct insulin consistently through the extra mucus and thickening produced by either of these problems.

So for the foreseeable future, the main way of delivering insulin to type 1 diabetics will be by injection. We have plenty of choice. There are many forms of insulin, and different ways of getting them through the skin, and each diabetic specialist has his or her own favourites. This book describes them, so that you can compare your own method with others. More important, it gives practical hints on how to achieve the optimum control of your diabetes by combining your eating and exercise habits (I hate to use the word diet) with the most effective insulin doses and delivery systems.

5

Eating

Eating wisely

To the general public the word 'diet' has, over the years, acquired a slightly pejorative ring. It has been mainly linked to the need for cutting down calorie intake in people who are overweight. Obese people 'go on diets' to lose weight, and it is obvious to anyone working with them that they usually fail. People switching to 'diets' may lose weight for a while, but the vast majority (the common figure quoted is 95 per cent) give them up and become just as obese as before within a year. So diets are seen as a temporary style of eating – one that is usually restricting in some way and often unpleasant or boring – that is used to achieve an aim and then cast aside when the aim is achieved.

We doctors and nurses use the word 'diet' for our diabetic patients in an entirely different way. We see it as a lifestyle to which people with diabetes must adhere permanently, and preferably very strictly. Not only is it a form of discipline, particularly for type 1 diabetics, it must also be organized in relationship to insulin injections and exercise habits. The three are interdependent and must not be thought of as separate.

Do not let this bald statement of the facts dismay you. Sticking to strict rules about food does not mean that eating is less enjoyable. In fact you may find that as you get used to the new habits food becomes much more enjoyable and tasty than before. One reason for that is that your new choices of food have more subtle tastes that are not drowned out by the addition of sugar (and, for that matter, salt, about which more later).

Take the story of Iain, the doctor described in Chapter 2 who developed diabetes after a mumps pancreatitis. Immediately after the diagnosis he stopped adding sugar to his tea and coffee. He had always had a sweet tooth, and thought that it would take time to lose it, but it didn't work like that. Within days he was enjoying the real tastes, not drowned in sugar or milk, of many different teas and coffees, and enjoying them thoroughly. He had no problem in abandoning desserts and sweets, baking and biscuits, cakes and scones because the substitutes, fresh fruits and vegetables, different types of bread, and different ways of cooking potatoes, pasta and rice, were much tastier and just as filling.

The other big change was in his timing of meals. Although he did not have to fit in his eating schedule with insulin injections (he was able to manage his mumps-induced diabetes without the need for insulin), he told me that it would have been easy to do so. Instead of his old habit of a light breakfast, a slightly more substantial lunch and a 'proper' meal in the evening, he quickly grew used to eating three moderate meals equally spaced throughout the day, making the last one a single course, finishing with a piece of fresh fruit.

He quickly realized that he enjoyed the radical change in his eating habits. He never ate so much that he felt full, he felt much less hungry during the daytime, and started to lose weight. Within two months he had lost his excess weight of around 13kg (2 stone), and he felt 'great'. He was no longer lethargic, had a much better sense of taste, had plenty of energy, was eating much less and was enjoying what he ate. More than 20 years later he is still eating in the same way, and considers himself lucky enough to have remained fit so far.

He claims that in no way could what he eats be called a 'diet' in the lay sense of the word, because it is enjoyable and not, to his mind, restrictive, although in the medical sense he had placed himself on a diabetic diet suitable to a type 1 diabetic. Its principles are discussed in more detail below.

Rules for healthy eating with diabetes: Iain's way of eating

First of all, everyone, diabetic or not, would benefit from eating in this way. So if you are the diabetic in your family, why not get your family and friends to enjoy this way of eating with you? It is difficult to be the only one in a family to be eating in one way, while all the others are tucking into fries, cakes and desserts. There is no need to buy special 'diabetic' foods, which are generally more expensive and not necessarily better for you. A generation ago, people with diabetes were restricted largely to salads and special breads and rolls that tasted like cardboard. Thank goodness we know better now.

Let's start on a positive note. If you like Italian, Greek and Spanish food, you'll like being on a 'diabetic diet' – because Mediterranean cooking is almost completely compatible with diabetes. But don't let it go to your head. It is important not to eat too much, whatever you are eating, because becoming overweight can put people with either type of diabetes at greater risk than others of heart attacks and strokes.

Eating rule 1: choose foods with a low glycaemic index

The first principle of eating well as a diabetic is to avoid foods and ingredients that, soon after they are swallowed, cause the blood glucose levels to rise steeply and therefore need a big surge of insulin to deal with the rise. These foods are defined as having a high glycaemic index ('glyc' relates to 'glucose', 'aemic' relates to 'haem' or 'blood'). The member of your diabetic care team who is responsible for looking after what you are eating, probably the dietician or the nurse, will have a comprehensive list of foods with a high glycaemic index. Suffice it to say here that they are mainly foods containing glucose, sugar or honey.

Some of these foods with a high glycaemic index, because they taste sweet, are obvious. Jam, marmalade, honey, sweets, chocolate, fruit squashes, tinned or preserved fruits, cakes, baking of any sort – these all have a high glycaemic index. But be careful about over-the-counter prepared foods. Look at the label and check if sugar or glucose features high on the 'nutritional information' section. You may be surprised to learn that baked beans, well known to be high in fibre (7.7g of fibre per 207g serving) is even higher in sugar (12.4g per 207g serving). That doesn't mean you shouldn't eat baked beans, but at least, when you are taking your whole day's food intake into account, remember the contribution that your baked beans has made to your carbohydrate intake, and be prepared to adjust your treatment accordingly. Better still, if you are desperate to eat baked beans, restrict them to a small amount.

Artificial sweeteners are very much in vogue. So-called diet fruit drinks are sweetened with saccharin and aspartame and other chemicals to make them more palatable to people who wish to retain their sweet tooth while slimming or are needing to control their diabetes. Many people also use sweeteners in their tea and coffee. I don't think that sweeteners help anyone. I don't have figures to prove my point, but my experience over many years has convinced me that people who keep up their taste for sweet foods by using artificial sweeteners always fall by the wayside and revert to their old sugary habits.

My patients who have deliberately decided to cut out all sweet-tasting foods (except for fresh fruit) have done much better and controlled their weight and their diabetes much more effectively. As proof of that, look into the trolleys of customers next time you are at the supermarket. I bet that the fat customers have several bottles of diet Coke or something similar in their trolley – and that the thin customers prefer the 'real thing' or confine their sweet purchases to fruit.

Diabetics who decide to cut out sweet foods can take comfort that it isn't socially unacceptable these days to refuse a dessert as a finish to a meal. It isn't as difficult to organize to cut out sweet foods as it is, say, to organize a diet for people with coeliac disease due to gluten allergy, or a diet for people with peanut allergy, or for vegans. If you have diabetes, a good strategy, when someone 'pushes' a sweet or a cake at you, is to explain that you have 'a little trouble with sugar'. That's always perfectly acceptable to the 'pusher' and the pressure disappears.

Another plus point about eating healthily in type 1 diabetes is that there is hardly ever any need to count calories. Once you have got used to your new eating habits, it is fairly easy to estimate how much, and what, to eat to fit with your usual insulin dose. It comes with experience and training, and soon is second nature, much like learning to ride a bicycle as a child.

Eating rule 2: space meals regularly throughout the day

The spacing of meals regularly throughout the day is the next main principle of healthy eating. Many people with no experience of diabetes in the family still stick to the old habits of hardly any breakfast and two main meals each day. One main meal is at lunchtime, and the other is in the early evening, nowadays seated around the television with a tray on the knee instead of around a table with the family. The pros and cons of this latest social change in eating habits are still heatedly debated, but what matters to type 1 diabetics is not where they eat, but what they eat, how much and how often.

It is important not to miss breakfast and to have three meals a day. If you stick to two large meals a day (and even more so if you stick to one), much of your intake will be sugars, and your blood glucose levels will rise so steeply that you will need large amounts of injected insulin to cope with them. It is far better for you to have three relatively small meals, with little refined sugar in them, at regularly spaced times throughout the day. Then you can co-ordinate the food more efficiently with your insulin injections, so that you can keep the doses you need relatively low.

A meal can mean anything from soup and a sandwich to meat, potatoes and vegetables, with a small dessert if you wish. Iain's decision not to eat desserts is his choice, and that doesn't suit everyone. What matters is that the load of food you eat at the meal coincides with the amount and type of insulin you have injected a few minutes beforehand. Some people with diabetes that is more difficult to control may need a snack between meals to keep their blood glucose level within the accepted limits. They may also need a snack last thing at night to avoid a hypo while asleep.

It is reasonable for people with type 1 diabetes to have the occasional treat – say a larger then usual meal while out, but if you do so, remember to increase your insulin dose just before the meal to avoid hyperglycaemia. Take the advice of your diabetic nurse or dietician about the size of the increase that you need with this type of meal.

Eating rule 3: eat plenty of starches

Although it's important to avoid sugars, it's just as important to eat plenty of starches, the other source of carbohydrate in food. The main sources of starch are potatoes, bread, pasta, rice and other cereals. It takes longer for starches than for sugars to be digested down to glucose in the gut, so that after a starchy meal, the blood glucose rise is much slower than after a sugary one. That means less insulin has to be given to bring the glucose into normal blood levels, so that the blood glucose curve after the meal is much closer to normal.

Even then, care should be taken in cooking. For example, boiled potatoes produce a much smaller and slower rise in blood glucose than baked potatoes. Wholemeal and multigrain breads, like boiled potatoes, have a low glycaemic index but white bread has similar glucose-raising properties to baked potatoes. The same goes for white rice and some breakfast cereals, such as cornflakes. Choose instead oat-based meal, such as porridge, and less refined cereals such as brown rice, bran-based breakfast cereals and muesli. When choosing your breakfast cereals keep these things in mind, and if you are in doubt, talk their properties over with your dietician and nurse.

Eating rule 4: remember roughage

Fibre has been going in and out of diet fashion for 40 years, since Dr Denis Burkett, working in east Africa, proposed that it protected against bowel disorders. The experts are still arguing about that theory, but there is no argument against the proposal that fibre is an essential ingredient of the daily food for type 1 diabetics. High-fibre foods have three advantages for people with diabetes:

- they reduce the rise in blood glucose after meals, so that less insulin is needed and the blood glucose curve is flatter;
- they help to lower blood cholesterol levels, a very important action for the long-term health of all diabetics, type 1 or type 2; and
- they tend to be very filling, so that they help you to eat less without leaving you hungry.

They also help people to lose weight and they help in producing normal daily bowel movements as well.

Fibre is the relatively indigestible material of plant stems and cell walls. We do not produce the enzymes to break them down in our gut (unlike herbivores like rabbits), so that fibre is not nutritious in itself, but it helps to slow down digestion of carbohydrates. This is the main reason for its ability to keep rises in blood glucose levels after meals to a minimum. Researchers have adopted this property to produce medicines, such as acarbose, about which there is more detail in the section on oral antidiabetic drugs (see Chapter 13).

Foods rich in fibre include multigrain bread, long-grain brown rice, wholegrain pasta, green and yellow vegetables (such as peas, beans, lentils, carrots, turnips, beetroot, cabbages, sprouts and lettuce) and unrefined wholegrain cereals.

Eating rule 5: don't overdo the fats

It is understandable that people are confused by the different messages on fatty foods. On the one hand we hear a lot about how damaging animal fats are to the heart and circulation. On the other we hear how beneficial vegetable oils (like sunflower oil and rape seed oil) and fish oils (from cod liver, halibut and oily fish in general) are. So should the type 1 diabetic do without dairy products and consume margarine instead?

There are two aspects of fats in food to be considered. The first, and of more immediate importance to people with diabetes, is that all fats, from whatever source, are a high source of calories. For example, 1g of carbohydrate (such as starch or sugar) provides 4 calories of energy, and 1g of protein (for example lean meat, poultry or fish) also provides 4 calories. However, 1g of fat or oil (of animal, fish or vegetable origin) provides 9 calories. Alcohol is close to fat in energy provision, in that 1g of pure alcohol gives you 7 calories.

So if you are fond of fries and oily foods, be aware that they are high-energy providers, and that you must take that into account in your diabetes control. Fats and oils are broken down into fatty acids by your digestive juices, to be taken up by the liver, which reorganizes them into the complex fats that the body needs (like cholesterol, about which much more later; see p. 74). These complex fats are distributed in three ways. Fats essential to the function of fat-rich organs (like the brain, the nerve cells of which are full of, and surrounded by, fat) are transported to these organs in the bloodstream. So a basic minimum of fat is essential in our food to keep organs like the brain and the liver, another organ that needs fats to function properly, healthy.

The problems arise when we eat too much fat for our needs. The excess is either stored in fat cells or converted to glucose and used to provide energy, in which, of course, insulin is involved. Excessive consumption of animal fats promotes the deposit of fat, in the form of cholesterol, in the walls of arteries, such as the coronary arteries supplying the heart or the cerebral arteries supplying the brain. There it causes inflammation and becomes the eventual focal points for the clots and haemorrhages that initiate heart attacks and strokes.

The process of laying down of fats in the blood vessel walls is accelerated in people with poorly controlled diabetes. They should therefore avoid over-consumption of animal fats, not just because they may become overweight and have trouble with their diabetes control, but also because they would be putting themselves at a higher than necessary risk of a heart attack or stroke. Vegetable and fish oils are different. They are less likely to lead to fatty deposits in the arteries, and there is good evidence that regularly eating foods rich in these oils actually protects you against heart attacks and strokes, because they promote the release of cholesterol deposits from the arteries.

So it should be good for you to eat oily fish (like mackerel, herring, tuna, sardines, pilchards, trout and salmon) around three times a week. Grill them, rather than fry them. When cooking, if you must enjoy a fry-up from time to time, use vegetable oils, but throw them away after they have been used twice. Preferably use fresh oil each time. This is because repeated heating of vegetable oils changes their composition so that they behave in your body more like animal fats.

Eating rule 6: keep slim

Your enthusiasm for oily fish and vegetable oils should not blind you to one of the most important messages for anyone with diabetes, type 1 or type 2: that is – do not allow yourself to become overweight. If you are already overweight, you must lose the excess pounds. For people without diabetes, being overweight is mostly just a nuisance. It is a cosmetic worry, perhaps, but as very many people in our society today are overweight, most people accept it and treat it as a minor problem that some day they may do something about.

For a diabetic that attitude would be a big mistake. Being overweight raises insulin needs and makes it much more difficult to control your blood glucose levels. It is also linked to higher than normal blood levels of the fats (low-density lipoprotein cholesterol and triglycerides, about which more later; see p. 74) that raise your risks of heart attacks and strokes. Obesity is linked, too, to high blood pressure, control of which is just as important as control of blood glucose (more about that later, too.

So, now that you have diabetes, you must take control of your own weight, and the only way to do that is to organize not just your eating habits and insulin injections but your exercise, too. If you are having trouble with your weight, then discuss your eating and exercise habits in detail with your dietician and diabetes nurse. They will together draw up a programme that combines the right way to eat and to exercise so that you will lose the extra pounds. Don't be tempted to follow those crazy low-calorie diets that are repeated again and again in women's magazines. They are not for diabetics (I would claim they are not for any normal person), and they could badly interfere with your diabetes control. Trust your medical and nursing team and stick by their instructions.

As for exercise, it isn't necessary to go running or to join a gym, although if you enjoy them, by all means do so. Simple walking is often good enough to lose weight. A half hour's brisk walking or swimming in the local pool, or an hour on a bicycle, every day will take a stone (7kg) off in a year, as long as you don't eat more. In fact, regular exercise often curbs the appetite, helping you to eat less. And after a week or so, you will begin to feel much better and fitter.

How do you know if you are overweight? That's simple. Just look in a long mirror. You can surely judge for yourself whether you have a spreading middle or hips. A man with a waist measurement of 39 inches (100cm) or more is considered to be overweight. The equivalent measurement for a woman is 36 inches (91cm). If you are above this level, you need to lose an inch or two, preferably more.

There is a more exact formula by which you can judge whether you are veering towards the obese: the body mass index (BMI). For the BMI you must know your weight in kilograms and your height in metres and centimetres. Divide your weight by the square of your height, and you should get a figure between 20 and 25, the normal range for BMI. Under 20 and you are a little too thin. Over 25 you are a little overweight. Over 30 you are fat enough to be diagnosed as clinically obese. Take my example. I'm 78kg (12 stone 7lb) and 1.78 metres (5 foot 10 inches); 1.78 squared is 3.17, so my BMI is 78 divided by 3.17, which is 24.6. That is just under the upper limit for normal, so I'm not overweight, but I still feel that it is slightly too heavy for me, so I'll take a little more exercise and eat a little less until I have lost 2–3kg (5–6lb) more. The BMI chart shown here will show you precisely where you relate to the norm, and how much weight you need to lose (or gain, if you are much underweight) to get into the normal range.

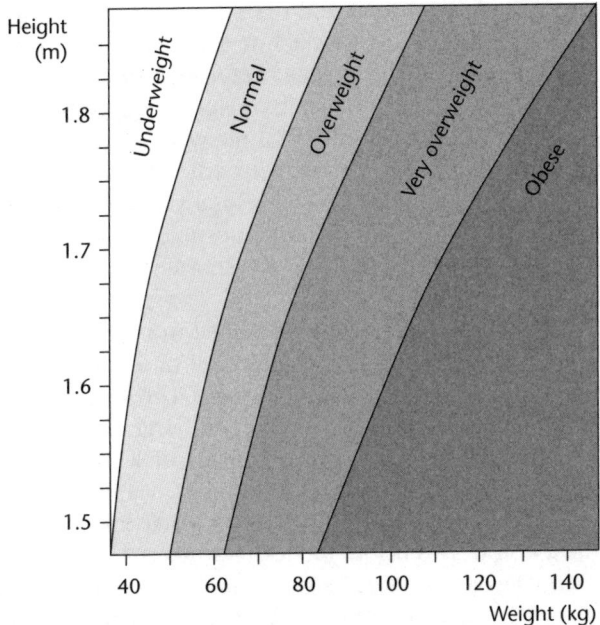

Figure 5.1 Body mass index (BMI) chart

One warning about the BMI. Well-muscled people may have a raised BMI yet still be lean, because muscle weighs more than fat. So the average BMI of an international rugby player would be well above the obese line, yet such a person would carry hardly an ounce of fat. These people are the exception, of course, but if you are in physical training and have increased your muscle bulk through exercise and weight training, then your BMI is a poorer guide to your fat deposits than it is for the average person.

Eating rule 7: use alcohol wisely

This is where you must discipline yourself especially strictly. Over the past few years the messages about alcohol have been confusing. In the early 1990s the idea of 'safe' amounts of alcohol was promoted, so that it became acceptable for men to drink 21 units a week and for women to drink 14 units a week without doing themselves any long-term harm. That came to be seen as that drinking up to that amount of alcohol was actually good for you – not the same message at all.

Then the red wine message hit the lay press. It came from a study by Professor Jean-Marc Orgogozo and his team at Bordeaux University.

I have met Professor Orgogozo, and I like him a lot. He is a good scientist, and is not funded by any special interest, such as the wine-makers. He started his research with the idea that regular drinking of red wine from a very early age, as happens in his region, might be harmful, so he followed drinkers and non-drinkers for many years, noting what they died from and at what age. He was astonished to find that the wine drinkers outlived the non-drinkers by several years, and the difference persisted when he removed all the other possible influences that might have prolonged the drinkers' lives (or shortened the non-drinkers' lives).

Clearly something in the red wine helped to protect drinkers from heart attacks and strokes. Was it the alcohol or a particular property of the wine unrelated to the alcohol as such? The academic argument continues: well-respected researchers in Edinburgh and Munich have reported similar effects in moderate drinkers of whisky or beer. The figures are confirmed by surveys of millions of deaths reported to life assurance companies, in which it is certain that lifelong teetotallers tend to die a year or two before moderate drinkers.

So is a little alcohol each day a good thing for people with diabetes? Much depends on what you define as a little, and whether you can keep it to a little. The standard advice is to drink no more than 2–3 units of alcohol a day if you are a woman and 3–4 units if you are a man. A unit means a single measure (25ml) of spirits (a 'half' in Scotland), a standard glass of wine, a small glass of fortified wine like sherry or port, and a half pint (250ml) of beer (even less than that if it is a strong beer).

However, this advice is for the general population, not type 1 diabetics. For you, the advice must be much more precise. To start with, alcohol is a high source of calories. (Remember that 1g of alcohol gives you seven calories, and that a single 25ml of spirits, for example, contains about 10g of alcohol.) Therefore you must take this into account when you are giving yourself your insulin. Secondly, too much alcohol drunk over even a moderate period can start to harm your liver, brain and peripheral nerves – the nerves that run between your limbs and the spinal cord and that detect sensations (pain, touch, heat, cold, vibration, position sense) and initiate muscle action. If you regularly overdo your alcohol intake you are inviting liver, brain and nerve disease, and once such damage has been established, it is hard to reverse.

If you already have signs of peripheral neuropathy (your specialist will probably already have done the necessary tests for it), even moderate amounts of alcohol can make it worse. A relatively minor loss of sensation in the fingers and toes can develop into constant pins and needles, numbness and inability to tell when water is scalding hot or freezing cold. And as peripheral nerves run to and from the genital area, one sign of diabetic neuropathy is impotence. Alcohol ruins the performance even of non-diabetics (read the gatekeeper scene in *Macbeth*): if you have type 1 diabetes the combination of alcohol and neuropathy can leave you impotent long after the hangover has gone.

So it is wise for all type 1 diabetics to keep their alcohol intake down to the minimum, say 1 or 2 units a day at most, and to have several days a week alcohol-free. If you already have neuropathy, seriously consider if you can do without alcohol altogether.

However much you drink, make sure that you never do it on an empty stomach. Paradoxically, alcohol on an empty stomach and not mixed with a sugar-containing drink can drive your blood glucose level down into the hypo region. If you must have a pre-meal drink, then have a starch-rich snack with it, such as a sandwich. That's important, too, at bedtime, if you like a small 'nightcap'. Don't have the drink on its own – have a savoury biscuit or a small sandwich with it. Otherwise you may have a hypo during the night, with its accompanying nightmares and restlessness and headache in the morning.

6

Organizing your insulin

Types of insulin

Insulin injections are classified by how fast they begin to act, and for how long they continue to act, after the injection. So they can be very fast acting, short acting, intermediate acting and long acting. They are also classified according to their origins. Until recently insulins have been prepared from extracts of animal pancreas: the early insulins taken from cows were known as beef insulins and the later ones, which almost always came from pigs, were known as porcine insulins.

Each animal species produces its own specific insulin, slightly different chemically from all the others. Porcine insulin is chemically closer to human insulin than beef insulin, and it is thought to cause fewer allergic reactions. Human insulin is either porcine insulin chemically modified to mimic the chemistry of human insulin or a synthetic insulin made by the latest in DNA technology, details of which are outside the scope of this book. One form of human insulin, for example, is made from an insulin 'precursor' chemical found in yeast cells.

Just because human insulin is the same substance as is produced by human beings does not mean that it is necessarily better at controlling your blood glucose than porcine insulin is. When it was first made available, many people who were switched to it from porcine insulin found that they didn't get on with it so well. Some found, for example, that they lost the warning signs of hypo attacks. That led to sudden loss of consciousness in some people who had not had hypos for years.

That period is thankfully behind us. Staff in diabetic clinics and general practice are well aware of the advantages and pitfalls of the different forms of insulin, and are able to give personal advice to every type 1 diabetic that is tailored to the individual and to his or her particular insulin needs. So you may be given porcine or human insulin: what matters is not the type you are prescribed, but whether it does the job with the least side effects for you. And the job is to maintain your blood glucose level as close to normal as possible.

Very rapidly acting insulins

Very rapidly acting insulins, such as aspart, glulisine and lispro, act faster even than soluble insulins. They are all human insulin analogues, and they start to work on blood glucose levels within five to 15 minutes of the injection, so that they are usually given immediately before, during or immediately after a meal. Their main effect is at around two hours after the injection, and although there is still some glucose-lowering activity for up to six hours, their action is shorter than that of soluble insulins. That means that if they are given three times a day, blood glucose levels measured before meals are slightly higher, and after meals are slightly lower, than with equivalent doses of soluble insulin. If you tend to have 'hypos' before meals, or you eat in the late evening and get hypos during the night, these insulins are designed for you. Aspart and lispro are normally given by injection under the skin (subcutaneously) either just before or just after meals. They are also given into a vein (intravenously) in some diabetic emergencies (such as hyperglycaemic coma) or just before and during surgery.

Short-acting insulins

Short-acting insulins are soluble and look clear in the syringe. Hypurin is the porcine form: Actrapid, Humulin and Insuman are human forms. Given under the skin (subcutaneously), they begin to act between 20 and 30 minutes after injection. The peak effect is at around three hours, and the activity lasts for six to eight hours depending on the dose. In an emergency, such as diabetic coma, they are given into a vein (intravenously), when they produce the desired effect within five minutes, but it only lasts for half an hour at most. To control your blood glucose properly throughout the 24 hours of a day using only soluble insulin you would have to give yourself strictly spaced subcutaneous injections every eight hours. Intermediate- and long-acting insulins are one answer to this inconvenience.

Intermediate- and long-acting insulins

The action of insulin can be lengthened to between 12 and 36 hours by combining it with various proteins. Examples of these preparations include isophane insulin and insulin zinc suspension. They look cloudy in the syringe and need only be given once or twice a day, provided that they control blood glucose levels well at this frequency.

Subcutaneous injections of intermediate- and longer-acting insulins start working on your blood glucose within one to two hours, have their maximum effects at between four and 12 hours, and continue to act for between 16 and 35 hours. So some are given once a day, and some twice daily.

However, in normal people, insulin levels in the blood fluctuate widely in response to their meals. This can't be mimicked by either more frequent injections of short-acting insulins or by less frequent injections of longer-acting insulins on their own. What is needed is a mixture of the two – the short-acting ones for mealtimes, when you need the 'spike' of insulin, and the longer-acting ones for in between meals when you want to keep the blood glucose on an even keel with a steady supply of insulin.

So the manufacturers have provided 'biphasic' insulins, mixtures of insulins with different lengths of action, to fit in with your own pattern of blood glucose. They contain different proportions of short- and longer-acting insulins, so that you can adjust the speed of onset and the length of action of the insulin combination to suit you. Among them are biphasic insulin aspart, biphasic insulin lispro and biphasic isophane insulin. Soluble insulin and longer-acting insulins can usually be mixed in the same syringe – the exceptions being detemir and glargine insulins, which must be given separately.

The longer-acting insulins include:

- isophane insulin, which is insulin in a suspension of protamine that is often used to initiate twice-daily insulin therapy; many people mix it with soluble insulin themselves, but it is also available in a ready-mixed form as biphasic isophane insulin, biphasic insulin aspart and biphasic insulin lispro;
- insulin zinc suspension, which has a longer action than isophane insulin and is used in a similar way;
- protamine zinc insulin, which is given once a day with soluble insulin, though it has been largely replaced by the other mixtures because of problems of binding within the syringe when it is used with soluble insulin; and
- insulin glargine and insulin detemir, which are human-type insulins with long duration of action; both are normally given once daily, although detemir can be given twice daily.

Your diabetic medical and nursing team will work out with you what should be best for your particular eating patterns, lifestyle and weight. They will then monitor your progress closely, with regular blood glucose and HbA1c measurements, and fine-tune the dosage for a few weeks. When they think the control is as good as they and you working together can achieve, you can then settle into a normal routine of insulin injections with appropriate eating pattern and exercise.

Timing of insulin injections

The timing of insulin injections is crucial. With the exception of the three very rapid-acting human-type insulins, which as mentioned above should be given immediately before, during or immediately after a meal, insulin should be given 15–30 minutes before meals. Aspart, glulisine and lispro are helpful if the meal is unexpected or you do not know how much food there will be.

Giving an insulin injection too long before eating may give you a hypo, since the insulin acts before the new glucose from the food enters the bloodstream. This is particularly important if some of the injection is short acting. Giving insulin (apart from the three rapidly acting exceptions mentioned above) too close to the meal may allow the glucose from the food rising too high in the bloodstream before the insulin starts to work. So the timing should be just right.

Although it would be good to be able to return to the old days of a once-daily injection of a biphasic insulin (see above), it does not give good enough control. So most people have to give themselves several injections in the day. Exceptions to the multiple daily dose rule are people with type 2 diabetes (see Chapter 13), who need a longer acting insulin injection last thing at night so that their early morning blood glucose is near-normal.

Twice-daily biphasic insulin, given before breakfast and before the evening meal, may work well. Most people on twice-daily insulin need a higher dose in the morning than in the evening and must eat small snacks between meals and at night. There is a growing tendency today, however, for people to give themselves short-acting insulin doses before each meal – normally three times a day – and to combine that with a medium- or long-acting dose at bedtime. A few people add a small dose of medium-acting insulin mid-morning. This gives them the chance to change doses to cope with different meal sizes and exercise, and to be much more flexible from day to day in their mealtimes. It also lets them do without the between-meals snacks, though they should always take that last-thing-at-night snack to avoid night-time hypos.

It takes time to master all the details of which insulin you should have, at what dose and how often, and how to adjust all of these with changing mealtimes and exercise sessions, but it is worth it. Once you have done so, you will find that the better quality of life this mastery gives is worth the bother of the extra injections each day.

Giving the injections

The syringes

All syringes are now of the disposable plastic type, and most have the needles fixed to them. They are designed to be thrown away after a single use, but they can be used several times if they are looked after properly. Do not do this, however, before talking about it with your doctor or diabetic nurse, who will give specific advice on how to keep the syringe and needle scrupulously clean. The key is to place it back in its plastic cover without rinsing it in any way and to store it in the refrigerator until it is needed again. In any case, throw it away after it has been used five times, or before that if the needle is blunt.

Syringes come in 30, 50 and 100 unit sizes and may differ in their markings, so become expert in recognizing your dose. If the type or size of the syringe is changed, get very clear instructions from your diabetic nurse on the dose you need and how it appears on the syringe scale.

To draw the right amount of insulin into the syringe, first pull back the 'plunger' of the syringe so that it takes in air to the mark of the dose of insulin you are giving yourself. Then insert the needle through the top of the insulin bottle and inject the air into it. With the syringe pointing up vertically, the bottle upside down, and the tip of the needle below the liquid surface, withdraw the plunger slowly and the insulin should appear in the syringe without bubbles in it. If you do get bubbles, push the plunger in again until the bubbles escape and withdraw it again, so that it is bubble free. Then take the needle from the bottle. If you are taking both a short-acting and a long-acting insulin, draw in the clear insulin first, then the cloudy, into the same syringe, and inject it immediately.

Many people now use insulin pens. In Scandinavia, for example, more than 85 per cent of all insulin-using diabetics of either type use pens, rather than syringes. Pens either come with a cartridge of 150 or 300 units of insulin that you load into them, or are preloaded with insulin by the manufacturer. Preloaded pens are disposed of after the insulin is used up. In either form of pen you dial up your dose before the injection. The needles can be changed as they become blunt. If you use a pen, make sure you have a spare, in case you break it or lose it. It happens!

The injection itself

Whatever you use, pen or syringe, how and where to give the injection is important. We used to advise cleaning the skin first with spirit, using cotton wool or a swab. Now we know that is unnecessary. It is not only inefficient at sterilizing the skin (which was why people used to do it), but frequent swabbing the skin with spirit or alcohol toughens it so that it is harder to slip a needle through it, and it makes needles blunt faster.

The insulin should be deposited under the skin, not into it, but not so deep that it gets into the underlying muscle. So you should use needles that are the right length for you. The standard needles are 12mm (½ inch) long, but you may find shorter needles (8mm or ⅜ of an inch, 5mm or ¼ of an inch) more appropriate. Whatever the length of the needle, you should pinch up a piece of skin into a fold, then push the whole length of the needle into it, holding it at right angles to the body surface. Then press the plunger straight down in one movement, making sure that all the dose is delivered before quickly withdrawing the needle.

Use different sites in rotation for your injections, never repeating the injection in exactly the same spot. If you must use the same general area of skin twice in a row, at least make the second injection site more than 2.5cm (1 inch) away from the first one. Repeating an injection at the same spot can cause overgrowth of the tissues at that spot, a condition called lipohypertrophy. This may be to do with the fact that insulin can stimulate growth of tissues if repeatedly injected into the same spot.

In a Finnish study reported in December 2000 of 100 people with type 1 diabetes, 65 per cent had injection site complications, most of them with lipohypertrophy of the tissues under the abdominal skin. Most of these people continually used a very small area for their injections (not much bigger than a postage stamp, according to the investigating doctors), and most had relatively poor glucose control (HbA1c more than 8.5 per cent). Unbelievably, many of the Finns had injected through a buttonhole into their abdominal skin because it was convenient. They were getting repeated injections in exactly the same place.

Less often than hypertrophy, repeat injections in the same place may lead to hollowing out of the skin and the tissues underneath. This process, called atrophy, is due to shrinkage of the fatty tissues under the skin as a result of their constant exposure to high concentrations of insulin. It is thought to be less common than it was because insulins are purer than they used to be.

You will have your own preferred injection sites – they vary from the outer upper arm to the front of the thighs and the skin of the lower abdomen. Some people find that the insulin effect acts sooner if they use the upper arm rather than the leg, others find the abdominal skin more efficient. It is difficult to see why this should be, but you will find out the areas that suit you best as you vary the sites yourself.

Injections, despite what some diabetic specialists may say, are not painless. They sting a bit. But if you have a burning sensation or pain after an injection, or the site becomes red afterwards, you should tell your doctor or diabetes nurse. You may not be injecting yourself correctly or you may be developing an allergy to the insulin preparation you are using.

Pen devices licensed for use in the NHS in the UK include Autopen, HumaPen, NovoPen, OptiClik and OptiPen. Recently, 'needle-free' insulin delivery devices have been licensed, which use a thin jet of fluid forced through the skin under power to 'squirt' the insulin under the skin. They are an alternative for people who absolutely cannot bear the needles, but most regular needle users don't find the needles enough of a discomfort to think of transferring to the needle-free systems. The two marketed in the UK at the time of writing (2009) are mhi-500 and SQ-PEN.

Replacement and disposal

Two final points may seem obvious but are important.

First, when visiting the pharmacist for your new prescription of insulin, syringe, pen, device or needles, take your old ones with you, so that you are sure that the repeat prescription is exactly the same as the last one. Check the trade name of the insulin and its colour code and strength, check that the pen or syringe has the same dose markings on it and that the needles are the same as your usual ones. That will help to avoid errors in dosage, in type of insulin and in delivery. It can be so easy to be lulled into a routine, and fail to notice a subtle difference that is potentially dangerous.

Second, you must be fully aware of the need to dispose safely of all your used materials, including the lancets you use to take your blood samples. So you should have your own 'sharps' bin at home, and arrange for its safe disposal, either through your local surgery or with your local authority's disposal team. That is especially important if there are children in the house or regular visitors, and also if you have a chronic infection that may contaminate all the materials you are using.

7

Tackling type 1 diabetes: testing and targets

Not so long ago the only testing that type 1 diabetics did for themselves was for glucose in the urine. It involved sticking strips of paper into samples and watching the colour change. The results were given in terms of plusses – 0 if there was no glucose, + for a minor amount, ++ for a moderate amount and +++ for severe glycosuria (glycosuria simply being a medical term for glucose in the urine). People and their doctors were expected to judge how well controlled the diabetes was from diaries containing daily test results.

That has been consigned to the past, and rightly so, because the amount of glucose in the urine is at best a very rough guide to what is going on in the blood. Today we recognize that the only way to control diabetes correctly is to use blood glucose tests. That's why you are issued with blood glucose testing gear and are asked to fill in the results accurately day by day. It is a shame that you must add daily finger pricks to your insulin injections – diabetics must put up with a lot of episodes of discomfort to look after themselves, but it is very definitely worth it in the long run.

Skin-prick blood glucose testing

The first object of all skin-prick blood glucose testing is to obtain a fresh drop of blood easily without coaxing by pressure, from some skin site. Many manuals suggest the fleshy skin of the fingertips should be used. That can be very painful, and it is important to rotate the fingertips used to prevent a frequently used finger from becoming painful and even scarred. My own preference is the back of a finger, behind the nail. It is less sensitive to the pain and bleeds just as profusely as the fingertip. An ear lobe is a good substitute.

It is important to get plenty of blood welling up from the 'jab' with the lancet, as the strip used for testing must be thoroughly covered with the blood. If you have to squeeze the finger to get the blood out, you may not get an accurate result.

Whatever strip test is used, you must time exactly the moment the blood touches the strip. If you are using a meter (most people use meters today) the timer button must be pressed exactly on time. If you are instructed to wipe the strip free of blood, then you must time that accurately, too. Some meters do this automatically.

If you are in any doubt about how to use your meter or how to check that your blood glucose testing is accurate, go through it in detail with your diabetes nurse or doctor. Remember that if you get a 'funny' reading, it may be the meter that is wrong, not your blood glucose. If you suspect that you are getting wrong readings, use the check fluids provided with the machine as a comparison. It is a good idea, too, to have your machine tested regularly against standard blood samples in the laboratory.

When to test

All type 1 diabetics should measure their blood glucose levels at least once a day, and note it down in a daily diary for review by their diabetes nurses or doctors. This is the only way to know whether you are keeping your glucose levels as close as possible to the normal pattern. The tests should be done at different times each day, so that an overall picture can be presented. In effect it is a blood glucose curve whose points are collected over a month or so.

Why is this so important? The lower you keep your glucose levels, the better your chance of avoiding the major complications of diabetes – heart attack, stroke, kidney failure, blindness, diabetic gangrene, repeated infections and peripheral neuropathy.

Your target blood glucose levels

Non-diabetics have a fasting blood glucose level (taken first thing in the morning around 12 hours after the last food) of around 5mmol/l or, in American usage, 90mg/dl. After eating a meal, their normal insulin response prevents their blood glucose from rising above 8mmol/l (145mg/dl).

In untreated or poorly controlled diabetes blood glucose levels can rise well above 20mmol/l (360mg/dl). The aim of most diabetic clinics is to get their patients' blood glucose levels down to between 4 and 7mmol/l (70–125mg/dl) before meals and between 7 and 10mmol/l (125–180mg/dl) between one and two hours after meals. With figures like these, their HbA1c will almost certainly be below 7.5 per cent, a figure linked with relatively low risk of later strokes, heart attacks and kidney failure.

Although these levels are not quite as low as the figures in non-diabetics, they are fairly strict targets for people with diabetes, who do not start to feel unwell with 'hyper' symptoms (see p. 25) until their blood glucose levels are persistently above 14mmol/l (250mg/dl).

These strict targets are there for good reason: it is essential for all diabetics, of either type, to understand that they cannot judge how well their diabetes is controlled by how they feel. You may feel well, but in fact be badly controlled, and be open to severe health risks.

Having type 1 diabetes is different from having any other illness, because you become the manager of your own treatment. If you have read everything this far, you will have accepted that you must do everything you can to keep your blood glucose under control, 365 days and nights a year, and 366 in leap years. You, and only you, can do that. Your doctors and nurses can advise, but only you can put the treatment into practice.

Planning ahead

Your main problem is that your life may vary from day to day, and with it your insulin requirements. If you had a normal pancreas, it would do all the work for you, altering your insulin output perfectly according to the food you have eaten. But you don't have a normal pancreas: you have to do all its work for it.

Eating

So to repeat the eating advice given a few pages ago in Chapter 5, you must have three regular if small meals every day, and if necessary snacks between them and at bedtime. There is no harm in going out for a meal, as long as you plan beforehand. Take your blood glucose testing kit with you, and test after it. You will then know whether you have altered your pre-meal dose correctly, and whether you have to give yourself an extra dose of fast-acting insulin to counter a very high blood glucose level. It will also allow you to make a different change in your insulin injection the next time.

You should plan ahead like this in all conditions in which blood glucose is likely to rise abnormally, such as physical and emotional stress and infections. Don't wait for the glucose to go up steeply – foresee the difficulty and increase the dose accordingly. After that, measure your blood glucose and see if you adjusted the dose closely enough.

Exercise

Exercise poses the opposite problem. If you are planning strenuous exercise (like tennis, squash, fast walking, running or, as in Sir Steve's case, Olympic rowing) decrease your insulin dose. The change may be by as little as 4 units or by as much as half your usual dose: only you can know, from your own experience of doing so and checking your blood glucose levels afterwards. You may also need to take extra glucose beforehand and during the exercise, to make sure you don't develop a hypo. Taking extra glucose and less insulin are not alternatives but are complementary.

It is important, too, to understand which dose of insulin affects which blood glucose test. For example, if you are giving yourself two doses of insulin each day, the morning dose affects not only the blood glucose level at midday, but also the one just before the evening meal. If the evening pre-meal blood glucose level is too high (persistently above 7mmol/l), you may have to consider three insulin doses a day or a higher morning dose of longer-acting insulin. Similarly, the evening insulin dose affects the pre-breakfast blood glucose level the next morning. If that is too high, then you may need a larger evening dose of longer-acting insulin or to switch to a different regimen, with perhaps more frequent doses of different insulins. If you are not achieving pre-meal blood glucose levels at or below 7mmol/l or after-meal levels at or under 10mmol/l, you should discuss the possibility of better control with your diabetes team.

Summing up: blood glucose testing

To summarize: please do one or two blood glucose tests a day and note with them your insulin injections, what you have eaten and the exercise you have done. If your control is not as it should be, your doctor and nurse should be able, from these data, to help you to organize your insulin injections and your eating habits and exercise so that the control will improve. They won't mind you doing so, and they won't think you are wasting their time. Anything that can be done to improve your glucose control will put off the day that you develop more serious illness – and that will be a great saving in their time in the long run.

A word about smoking

A final thought in this chapter – in this book we have not yet mentioned smoking. People with either type of diabetes are mad to consider even smoking one cigarette a day. In Chapter 12, I explain why, if you do smoke, you must stop, and how to stop. For the moment, however, it is enough to state that smoking can foul up not just the lungs but also the lives of everyone, and especially of those with diabetes. So please don't smoke, ever. Just following that simple piece of advice could save your life.

8

Pumps and transplants

Sometimes even the best efforts at controlling type 1 diabetes with insulin injections are not good enough. For people with difficult-to-control diabetes (often called brittle diabetes), the bouts of hypos and hypers and the need always to be changing their doses, their eating habits and their social lives become overwhelming. They despair, and they can't cope with the distress and the serious side effects that their diabetes brings. They need something more than injections of insulin to help them overcome them. For them there are two extra approaches – insulin pumps and pancreatic transplants. Neither is undertaken lightly.

Insulin pumps

The principle of insulin pump treatment is that the patient has a continuously operating blood glucose sensor: this tells the pump how much insulin the pump needs to deliver to keep the glucose levels within the target range. The insulin used is rapidly acting, and the dose varies from minute to minute. The following review of pumps is based on the work of the team of Dr David Kerr, consultant physician, and Helen Nicholls and Janet James, nurse specialists, in the Diabetes and Endocrine Centre at the Royal Bournemouth Hospital.

They published a review of their work from 1998 in the April 2008 issue of *Practical Diabetes International*. It makes wonderful reading. They wrote that continuous subcutaneous insulin infusion (CSII) pump therapy for type 1 diabetes has four main benefits:

- improved blood glucose control;
- fewer blood glucose readings above and below target levels compared with the usual insulin injections;
- reduction of severe hypo episodes, particularly at night; and
- a consistent and invariable improvement in each patient's quality of life.

When might CSII therapy be recommended?

The Bournemouth results were part of the evidence examined by the National Institute for Clinical Excellence, now known as the National Institute for Health and Clinical Excellence (NICE), in their 2003 decision to recommend CSII therapy for patients with type 1 diabetes for whom the usual insulin injections (including insulin glargine) had failed, providing that the patients have the commitment and the competence to use it effectively. Failure of the previous treatment was defined as inability to maintain an HbA1c no greater than 7.5 per cent without disabling, repeated and unpredictable hypo episodes despite a high level of self-care.

CSII is offered only by a trained specialist team involving a physician interested in pump therapy, a diabetes nurse specialist and a specialist dietician. Patients entering the CSII system must be trained in its use and have strong ongoing support. At the Bournemouth Diabetes and Endocrine Centre, patients are educated in all these aspects of their management before they are accepted into CSII. They have online learning at <www.b-dec.co.uk> and home-based television communications with their hospital team. The Bournemouth team offer CSII to the usual adult type 1 patients and to children, adolescents, women wishing to become pregnant and pregnant women.

There are many other teams offering CSII around the country. If you feel you need this therapy, you must be very motivated to succeed, be realistic in your expectations, be willing to monitor finger-stick blood glucose levels at least four times a day, have good self-management skills and be very sure of the relationship between counting carbohydrate intake and insulin dose adjustments. The Bournemouth system now uses 'continuous interstitial glucose monitoring devices' – devices that are implanted under the skin to measure blood glucose automatically – with their pumps. These devices have been 'enormously beneficial' in solving problems such as the cause of night-time seizures related to hypos, in finding unacceptably high or low glucose levels even in people with a satisfactory HbA1c, and in reducing hyper peaks in pregnancy.

By 2008, the Bournemouth team had placed 112 patients aged from 20 to 92 on CSII. The average HbA1c levels of these patients have dropped from 8.73 per cent to 7.96 per cent – a big improvement in patients with such difficult-to-control diabetes. The patients reported that they are able to correct abnormal glucose levels much more easily using small changes in insulin doses, and the team report fewer episodes of ketoacidosis, fewer problems with infusions and fewer infections, especially in young adults.

In the 2008 article, Dr Kerr wrote that the 'availability of insulin pump therapy and continuous glucose monitoring systems is still patchy across the UK'. I'm sure that this will change very rapidly in the next few years.

Pancreatic transplants

The great hope for the future is to be able to transplant beta cells from a pancreas into patients with type 1 diabetes for whom all other treatment has failed. Naturally, such a programme has many theoretical and practical pitfalls. We have to transplant enough insulin-producing cells to make a significant difference to the abnormal glucose levels; they have to survive inside the alien environment of another person's immune system, and they have to continue to produce insulin for years.

Two possible approaches involve either transplanting pancreases as a whole or in part, or simply growing pancreatic beta cells in laboratory culture and transplanting them. It's estimated that we need only a quarter of a normal pancreas and that it is feasible to grow enough beta cells to maintain glucose levels near enough to the normal pattern. In essence, this would 'cure' diabetes.

Naturally the research is full of problems. Getting good enough pancreatic tissue, and growing viable and functioning beta cells, has proved elusive and difficult, but neither has proved to be impossible. I'm so grateful to be acquainted with one young woman who is the best example of the benefit of transplant I know. She has given me permission to tell her story.

Julie
Julie was in her late teens when she developed type 1 diabetes. It was severe from the start. Despite the best efforts at control by herself and her diabetes team, she had many episodes of hypos and hypers, and she quickly developed both retinopathy and nephropathy. As her kidneys and eyesight failed, she was put on dialysis and had numerous sessions with laser treatment for her sight. With her first pregnancy her health deteriorated further, and we despaired that she would ever see her son grow up.

She was on the kidney transplant list, and it was decided to perform a pancreas and kidney transplant at the same time. Imagine our joy when both the organs 'took'. For the first time in years she could pass urine and could do without her injections. Much more than that, her retinopathy, which we thought must be irreversible, began to improve. So for the first time in years, too, she could see well enough to drive.

It is now ten years since her double transplant. She and her son are well and happy together. She is still driving. No one who knew her when she was at her worst can believe that she is the same woman.

If only we could do the same for the many hundreds of young women and men who are in the same position as Julie was. Transplants, because of their difficulties and costs, are always going to be a last resort and for severe diabetes, but they will surely become more commonplace as the problems are solved. My feeling is that the use of 'bags' of beta cells (grown in the laboratory, they will be inserted into the abdomen inside membranes that will prevent the immune system from attacking the cells and causing rejection) is more likely to be the way forward than pancreatic transplants. I'm looking forward to seeing which method will take precedence in the next few years.

9

Type 2 diabetes

If you have type 1 diabetes, you may be tempted to skip the next two chapters, which concentrate on the other main form of the disease, type 2. Please don't. Although the initial symptoms and the underlying cause of your difficulties with blood glucose are different, you share very similar problems of self-management and a similar range of complications. So I make no apology for including a section on type 2 diabetes in a book for people with type 1 diabetes. Besides, most people I know with insulin-dependent diabetes are curious about the type 2 disease and about why one form of the disease always needs insulin injections while the others can usually 'get away' without them. It is sometimes a sore point for them! These chapters explain why.

A history: the Pima Indians and the Nauruans

In the early 1900s the Pima Indians living in the semi-desert lands of the south-western USA were a healthy people. They were poor and only just managed to scrape a living, but photographs taken at the time show them to have been slim and fit. By the 1960s they were a very different people. With the coming of industry and the loss of their traditional lifestyles, the grandchildren of those early twentieth-century native Americans grew up to be obese men and women, half of whom have type 2 diabetes. Instead of the so-called civilized world bringing them better health and longer life, they are dying much earlier than their grandparents from strokes, kidney failure and heart attacks. These were illnesses that were, along with their diabetes, virtually unknown to their grandparents. The Pima who remain physically active, stick to their old ways, or stay slim do not develop diabetes and do not die early.

The Pima are not alone. While they were developing their type 2 diabetes, exactly the same was happening on the other side of the world to the Nauruan islanders of the south Pacific. Today's Nauruans are much fatter than their ancestors, and they have paid a very heavy price in that half now have type 2 diabetes and the heart attacks and strokes that go with it.

The tragedies of the Pimas and the Nauruans are well known to medical students and doctors interested in diabetes all over the world, and their stories led to much greater understanding of the processes that lead to type 2 diabetes. The lessons learned from studying them have become a model for its treatment. They showed that the main danger in type 2 diabetes is not the disease itself, but its complications. As with type 1 diabetes, it is easy to get by with reasonable control of the blood glucose, but the real skill is to keep the patient well into old age.

Why did lifestyle changes cause an increase in type 2 diabetes?

Why should type 2 diabetes be so common in the American Indians and the Nauruans? The clue may lie in the fact that only two generations ago, they both survived by hunting and gathering food, and had to store fat in their tissues (mainly around the waist in men and around the hips in women) in times of plenty so that they could live on it and survive when food was scarce. In 1962, Dr J. V. Neel, writing in the *American Journal of Human Genetics*, suggested that there was an advantage to hunter–gatherers if their insulin activity directed more glucose to be stored in the fat and less in the muscles when they had plenty to eat. Their muscles would take up substantial amounts of glucose only when they needed it – for example actually during the hunt, when they were expending a lot of energy in running.

In 1998, Dr G. M. Reaven took this theory further. He proposed that muscle proteins (the chemicals that make muscles contract and relax) are conserved better when there is less glucose around the muscle fibres. Hunter–gatherers who need more than the usual amounts of insulin to drive glucose into their muscles, and whose muscles take up glucose from the bloodstream only when they are exercising hard, may have healthier and stronger muscles than those with normal insulin–glucose responses.

So this insulin resistance, in which you need a much higher than usual insulin level in the blood to drive glucose levels into the muscles (and therefore to bring down blood glucose levels) is an advantage for the hunter–gatherer. But it becomes a big disadvantage when the hunter–gatherer gives up his active lifestyle, becomes a near-couch potato, and starts eating more. His genetics remain the same, so he creates more and more fat stores, his blood glucose remains high (because without exercise it takes a lot more insulin than in the rest of the population to bring it down) and he becomes obese. At the same time, his blood pressure rises, the excess fats in his bloodstream start to damage his circulation, and he becomes much more prone to heart attacks and strokes.

In the last few paragraphs I have used the male pronouns because hunters were usually male. But the gatherers were women, and their lifestyles as the partners of the hunters were at least as strenuous physically, and often more so. For them, too, insulin resistance offered advantages in times of food scarcity and high physical activity. So female Pima Indians and Nauruan islanders inherited the same pattern of insulin resistance as their male counterparts. Now that they, too, have more sedentary lives and have an abundance of food to eat, half of them similarly have type 2 diabetes.

Differences between type 1 and type 2 diabetes

This background is quite different from the process that causes type 1 diabetes. If you have a tendency to develop type 1 diabetes, your pancreas has started off normally producing insulin, and rising glucose levels in the blood respond normally to it. As long as the pancreas continues to produce insulin, the relationship between insulin and glucose remains normal, so that the glucose in the blood is transferred in the usual way into the muscles, brain and all other tissues and organs.

Causes

Your type 1 diabetes started when some process caused your insulin production to fail. We are still not sure what that process is. It seems to be an autoimmune change, in which the body's immune system begins to mistake a protein produced normally by the body for a 'foreign' protein (as if it were the protein of an invading organism like a virus or a bacterium, or an abnormal protein from a cancer cell). Once that occurs, the immune system destroys the protein (in this case insulin) and the cell system that makes it (in this case the beta cells of the pancreas).

So in type 1 diabetes, your problem lies in the inability of the pancreas to produce the insulin that you need, because the cells that normally produce insulin have been destroyed by your body's own immune system.

There is no such problem in type 2 diabetes. To begin with, the pancreas produces plenty of insulin. In fact it may over-produce it, so that blood levels of insulin are higher than normal. But even with this excess of insulin production, blood glucose levels remain slightly higher than normal, because the insulin 'pump' cannot drive the glucose from the blood into the tissues, where it should be used for energy, or back into the liver, where it should be stored as glycogen.

So to start with the person with type 2 diabetes usually has relatively high blood glucose levels and high insulin levels, too. The beta cells of the pancreas work overtime to produce more and more insulin to try to drive the glucose levels down, but eventually they give up the struggle, and the production of insulin falls. That is when the diabetes starts in earnest. The blood glucose levels become so high that they reach the levels seen in type 1 diabetes, and much less insulin than normal is produced in response to a glucose-containing meal.

However, the underlying biochemical differences between type 1 and type 2 diabetes may not be so clear cut as the above explanation suggests. It used to be thought that there were distinct age differences between people with type 1 and type 2 diabetes. Type 1 diabetes was thought to start almost exclusively in childhood or during the teenage years and type 2 diabetes in the middle aged and older – hence the old terms of 'juvenile' diabetes and 'maturity-onset' diabetes mentioned in Chapter 2. The classical old division of treatments for the two types of diabetes is reflected in the other names for them – type 1 as insulin-dependent diabetes and type 2 as non-insulin-dependent diabetes.

These two classifications (juvenile versus maturity-onset diabetes and insulin-dependent versus non-insulin-dependent diabetes) are less used in expert circles now, because teenage cases of type 2 diabetes are becoming commoner, and because many type 2 diabetics need insulin to give them the optimum control of their blood glucose levels. To muddle things further, in 1993, Dr T. Tuomi, Professor Paul Zimmet and their colleagues reported finding autoimmune antibodies against the production of insulin in between 10 and 15 per cent of older people labelled as type 2 diabetics. These people were considered to have an 'incomplete type 1 autoantibody process' and an illness with the symptoms and properties of type 2 disease.

Onset and diagnosis

Whatever the technical aspects underlying the disease, people may possess the elements of type 2 diabetes for years before the imbalance between insulin and glucose levels (medically it is called insulin resistance) becomes bad enough to give obvious symptoms. The start of type 1 diabetes in childhood is a rapid change in previously healthy children or teenagers. They become severely ill in a matter of days, with rapid weight loss, severe thirst and a great increase in the volume of urine, night and day. There is usually little doubt about the diagnosis within days of its onset.

In stark contrast, the onset of type 2 diabetes is almost always very gradual. Typical type 2 patients have put on, rather than lost, weight. They have taken little exercise: they probably have not done enough regular exercise to make them healthily breathless for some years. But when they have had to run for a bus or climb some stairs, they do get a bit 'short of breath'. They usually put that down to their age and excess weight, but do little about it. It is only when they notice that they are sleepier than they used to be, say, in the middle of the day, especially after meals, and that they have started to get up at night to pass urine, and that they may be drinking a bit more than before, or that they are not seeing as well as they used to, that they ask to see their doctors.

They may not even do that. Many people with type 2 diabetes are found because they have other, apparently minor, problems that their doctors suspect are diabetes-related, like repeated skin or other infections, such as boils or thrush (high blood glucose levels leave you more than usually susceptible to repeat infections). Other cases are found on routine examinations, say for life insurance, or at 'well woman' or 'well man' clinics. Some are sent to their doctors by opticians, who have detected, on a routine test for glasses, early cataract or changes in the retina (in the back of the eye) that point to diabetes.

Looking back afterwards, especially when they have started treatment for their diabetes and begin to feel better, they usually realize that they have been 'under par'. However, most people like this have put their minor malaise down to their 'age' or 'stress', and are surprised by the diagnosis.

To summarize: the classic symptoms of type 2 diabetes are the gradual onset of thirst along with the need to pass more urine, day and night; tiredness, skin infections including thrush in the throat or in the vagina, in a person who is usually, but not always, overweight. However, because the symptoms have taken so long to develop fully, many people ignore them, or put them down to age and middle-aged spread.

Partly because of this attitude, for every person in a developed country known to have type 2 diabetes there is at least another with it who is yet to be diagnosed. In the UK, for example, where there are more than half a million known type 2 diabetics, there are another half million at least with the disease but who do not know it. Just as importantly, neither do their doctors. Not only that, but half the people known to have type 2 diabetes have no symptoms of it at all. They were diagnosed fortuitously when their urine was examined at a routine examination, and sometimes they resent having to be labelled with the disease and to change their lives accordingly.

That resentment, though understandable, is misplaced and can even be dangerous if they deduce from their lack of symptoms that type 2 diabetes is a mild disease and they need not change their lifestyle. On the contrary it is a serious health problem, that is just as likely to cause early death from heart attacks, strokes and kidney failure as type 1 diabetes, so even if you feel well without treatment, you must keep it under strict control. If you do keep it under control, you can reduce your chances of an early heart attack, stroke or kidney failure by more than 50 per cent – and that is enormously worth your while.

Control of diabetes

People with type 2 diabetes monitor their diabetes in a similar way to those with type 1 diabetes – by their blood glucose tests. These tests are used to make the diagnosis in the first place, and to judge progress thereafter.

Diagnosis of diabetes

There are two different protocols for the diagnosis of type 2 diabetes, one produced by the World Health Organization (WHO) and one produced by the American Diabetes Association (ADA). The WHO advises that diabetes should be diagnosed if the fasting plasma glucose (first morning glucose level after a night without food) is more than 7.8mmol/l or a random plasma glucose level (a test taken at any time of day) is above 11.1mmol/l. If the fasting plasma glucose is between 6.0 and 7.8mmol/l, or the random plasma glucose is between 7.8 and 11.1mmol/l, then an oral glucose tolerance test should be done. This means the person swallows 50g of glucose, and blood samples are taken for two hours afterwards. If after two hours the plasma glucose is above 11.1mmol/l, diabetes is diagnosed. If it is between 7.8 and 11.1mmol/l, the patient has 'impaired glucose tolerance' – a halfway stage between normal and diabetes. If it is below 7.8mmol/l, then the person is considered to be normal. People with fasting plasma glucose levels below 6mmol/l or random plasma glucose levels below 7.8mmol/l are considered non-diabetic.

In 1997 the ADA advised its doctors to rethink how to diagnose types 1 and 2 diabetes. The first was re-classified as type 1 (beta cell defect, usually autoimmune) and the second as type 2 (insulin resistance with an insulin secretory defect). Type 2 diabetes was to be diagnosed entirely from a fasting plasma glucose level (taken first thing in the morning 12 hours after the last food) of 7.0mmol/l or more. There were to be no oral glucose tolerance tests. If the fasting plasma glucose was between 6.0 and 7.0mmol/l then the patient was diagnosed as having impaired glucose tolerance. A fasting plasma glucose under 6.0mmol/l meant no diabetes.

Several points should be made here. One is that plasma glucose (the amount of glucose in a blood sample after the red cells are removed) is the routine way that blood glucose levels are measured in laboratory machines, and are usually slightly higher than those in whole blood (which still contains the red cells), which is what is used in finger-prick testing. The other is that the difference between the Americans and WHO in the way the diagnosis is made has not yet been resolved. However, the American method saves a lot of time in coming to decisions and costs in extra tests, and has been adopted by most countries and specialists.

What it also does is to give targets at which every type 2 diabetic can aim. If they can manage to keep their fasting plasma glucose under 7.0mmol/l (this is equivalent to a finger-tip blood level of around 6mmol/l), they are doing very well.

Beyond blood glucose ...

However, in both type 1 and type 2 diabetes the priority is hardly ever just about keeping your blood glucose in check. In many patients with either form of diabetes it is often part of a much more complex series of problems. Many people with type 2 diabetes, for example, are now given the label 'metabolic syndrome' (see Chapter 10). If you have diabetes of either kind, you must face up to every aspect of these problems if you wish to give yourself the best chance of surviving into a healthy old age. Type 2 diabetics could probably solve their problems by becoming hunter–gatherers like our ancestors, but that might be socially unacceptable. Nevertheless they can still do a lot for themselves by indulging in plenty of physical exercise and eating healthily, and seeking medical help. How doctors found out the best way to provide that help is described in the next chapter, which describes the work of the United Kingdom Prospective Diabetes Study.

10

The metabolic syndrome

Type 2 diabetes used to be thought of as the 'mild' form of the disease. After all, most people with it didn't have to take insulin injections. They didn't develop ketoacidosis, they didn't lapse into comas and they were less likely to become blind, or develop kidney failure, than those with type 1 diabetes. So as long as their blood glucose levels were reasonably controlled, it was assumed that they would sail on in life without much trouble. True, they did tend to have heart attacks and strokes a bit earlier in life than expected, but there was no proof that controlling their blood glucose more strictly would make any difference to that. And as most people with type 2 diabetes felt reasonably well there did not seem much point in striving for better control, particularly as it might put them at risk of 'hypo' attacks.

The components of the metabolic syndrome

High blood pressure and protein in the urine

These attitudes to type 2 diabetes started to change in the 1960s, largely as the result of work done by Professor Harry Keen, Professor of Human Metabolism, and his team at Guy's and St Thomas' Hospital in London. Professor Keen pointed out in the 1960s that there were 'bad companions' to diabetes, in persistent high blood glucose levels, high blood pressure (hypertension) and microalbuminuria (the appearance of microscopic amounts of protein in the urine, a sign of early kidney disease). All of these, he proposed, were mainly responsible for people with type 2 diabetes dying early from strokes, heart attacks and kidney failure.

Professor Keen and his colleagues were far-sighted. It was largely as a result of their basic work on the long-term damage that type 2 diabetes does to people that the United Kingdom Prospective Diabetes Study (UKPDS) was set up in the 1970s. The UKPDS made its reports in 1998, and it established not only the extent of the illnesses and deaths caused by type 2 diabetes, but also how they could be best prevented.

Abnormal blood lipids

On the way to these results, UKPDS added two more elements common to the cause of illness in type 2 diabetes – abnormal blood lipid (cholesterol) levels and smoking. In 1988, Dr G. M. Reaven named the combination of high blood glucose levels, high blood insulin levels, high blood pressure, high blood cholesterol levels and microalbuminuria as 'syndrome X'. He showed that people with this combination of problems had a very high risk of heart attack and stroke much earlier in life than would be normally expected, and suggested that all the factors that contributed to syndrome X be treated very vigorously to try to reduce that risk.

Overweight

However, Professor Reaven's description was incomplete. One more illness-creating sign had to be added – central obesity. That is, people who were overweight in a particular way, who put on extra fat around their waists, rather than round their buttocks and hips, and who possessed all the other syndrome X factors too, were in particular danger. In effect, the apple-shaped person was at more risk than the pear-shaped!

The complete picture

The complete picture, then, combining all these signs and symptoms, is now known as 'metabolic syndrome'. UKPDS showed that most people with type 2 diabetes have metabolic syndrome to some degree. In fact, their high blood pressure, their abnormal blood lipids, their apple-shaped obesity and even their microalbuminuria were probably all present up to ten years before they developed obvious type 2 diabetes. Their 'signpost' to future diabetes would have been a slightly raised fasting blood plasma glucose level (between 6 and 7mmol/l) and raised insulin levels. These figures are not enough to make the diagnosis of diabetes, but they can be called 'pre-diabetic', and people in whom these results are found, especially if they are also overweight and have high blood pressure, must be treated exactly as if they are already diabetic. Their risks of strokes and heart attacks are already rising – and they should be minimized.

In effect, these people must keep their blood glucose, their blood pressure and their blood cholesterol levels under control. How to do this is what the rest of the book is about. It may sound complex, but really it isn't. If you have type 2 diabetes you may even enjoy the challenge, and if you succeed you could well add 20 healthy and active years to your life expectancy.

The UKPDS studies confirmed how necessary it is for anyone with diabetes to follow the rules. If you want to keep as healthy as you can, and avoid deteriorating eyesight, the possibility of kidney failure and the probability of a heart attack or stroke, then you must keep strict control of both your blood glucose and your blood pressure.

But you must also not lose sight of the other risks – your cholesterol, your weight and, if you are mad enough to smoke, your smoking habit. The next few chapters will help you to control them, too.

11

Being in control

If you have read this book from the beginning you will already have got the repeated message – you must be in control of your own life if you are to survive into a healthy old age. Let us assume that you have just been diagnosed as having diabetes. How do we continue from this point?

The first thing is to find out how severe it is, and how many of the risk factors for early death from heart disease and diabetic complications you possess. That is done quickly and easily. You will be weighed and measured, and your waist measurement will be taken – so you will learn how obese you are, and what type of obesity it is.

Your blood pressure will be taken, as will your random blood glucose level, and a time to return for a fasting blood glucose level will be arranged. Just as important, you will have a blood lipid profile done, to check on those all-important low-density lipoprotein (LDL) and high-density lipoprotein (HDL) cholesterol levels, and your urine will be examined for microalbuminuria. Within a few days, all the results will be back, and your doctor will have a plan of treatments to correct anything that needs correcting.

Getting the weight right: eating healthily

Let's take the different aspects of treatment one by one, starting with weight. If you are overweight, then you absolutely *must* lose *all* the extra pounds. This isn't the same advice on weight as is given to non-diabetics who are overweight – most of them can be a few pounds over with no real risk attached. For you, being slim is a necessity. If you can lose those extra pounds, you may at the same time lose a lot of your other problems – your high blood pressure, your high blood glucose levels, your abnormal cholesterol profile, the lot. So go to it. Try to become that hunter–gatherer that you really should be, at least in shape and energy, if not in lifestyle.

You know your height, so aim for a weight that brings your BMI into the middle range of normal – say 22.5. And be sensible in the way you go about it. You will surely have to abandon the eating habits that made you overweight in the first place. The diabetic team looking after you is bound to have a dietician or a diabetes nurse trained in teaching healthy eating habits to diabetics. So make an appointment, and get learning.

The principles of what you must do are easy. You eat plenty of starchy carbohydrates and fibre, plenty of fresh fruit, moderate amounts

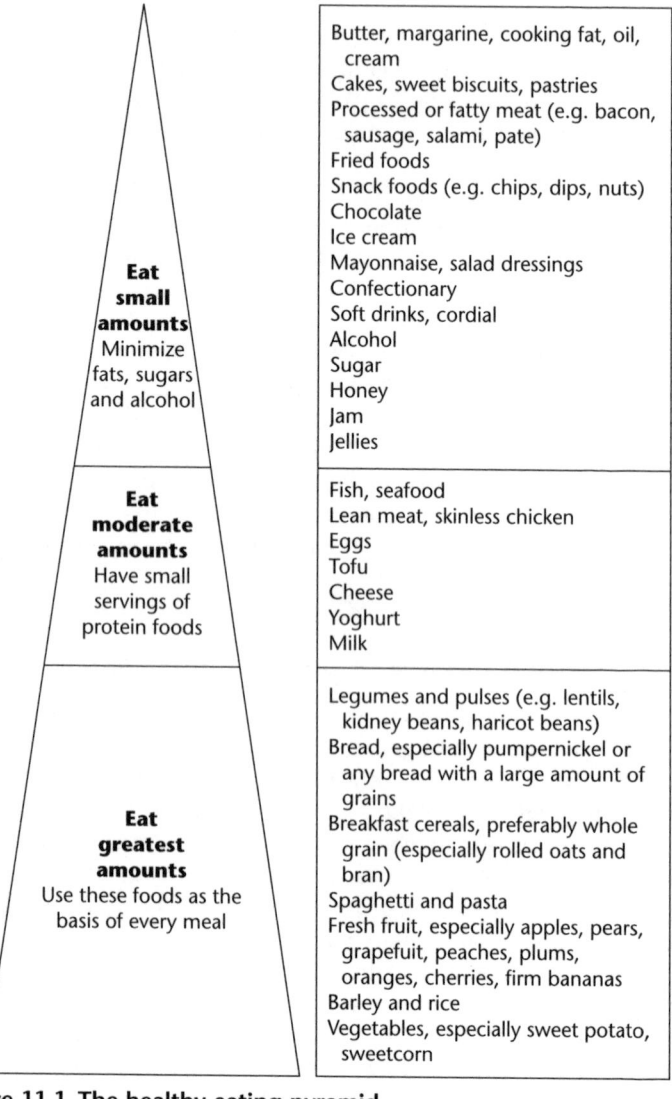

Eat small amounts
Minimize fats, sugars and alcohol

Butter, margarine, cooking fat, oil, cream
Cakes, sweet biscuits, pastries
Processed or fatty meat (e.g. bacon, sausage, salami, pate)
Fried foods
Snack foods (e.g. chips, dips, nuts)
Chocolate
Ice cream
Mayonnaise, salad dressings
Confectionary
Soft drinks, cordial
Alcohol
Sugar
Honey
Jam
Jellies

Eat moderate amounts
Have small servings of protein foods

Fish, seafood
Lean meat, skinless chicken
Eggs
Tofu
Cheese
Yoghurt
Milk

Eat greatest amounts
Use these foods as the basis of every meal

Legumes and pulses (e.g. lentils, kidney beans, haricot beans)
Bread, especially pumpernickel or any bread with a large amount of grains
Breakfast cereals, preferably whole grain (especially rolled oats and bran)
Spaghetti and pasta
Fresh fruit, especially apples, pears, grapefuit, peaches, plums, oranges, cherries, firm bananas
Barley and rice
Vegetables, especially sweet potato, sweetcorn

Figure 11.1 The healthy eating pyramid

of protein, and a minimum of fats, sugary foods and alcohol. You eat small meals regularly, rather than one or two large meals a day. For the fine details, however, you need to learn how to make meals appetizing, so that you actually like what you are eating, and even enjoy preparing the food. For that, depend on the dietician for hints and ideas. He or she can advise on all sorts of different cuisines, including ethnic cooking, and tailor them to your needs.

Take family members along to the meeting with the dietician if you can, particularly if they are involved in the cooking. It is just as important for them to know what you should be eating as it is for you. As everyone would benefit from the type 2 diabetes style of eating, it will do them good if they eat along with you. It isn't easy to be the only one in the family eating healthily while the rest are stuffing themselves with beef burgers and chips, puddings, custard and ice creams.

I like to use the healthy eating 'pyramid' devised by Professor Paul Zimmet and Dr Matthew Cohen of the International Diabetes Institute, Victoria, Australia, as a help to people wanting a quick check on what to eat most, what to eat in moderation, and what to eat least. It is reprinted here from the *Clinician's Manual on Non-Insulin Dependent Diabetes Mellitus*, published by Science Press in London.

People with type 2 diabetes can be more flexible in their eating habits than those with type 1, who need to correlate their eating with insulin injections. But they still need to eat their three meals a day, particularly if they are using hypoglycaemic drugs (about which more later; see p. 91). If you miss a meal while taking them you risk having a hypo.

Getting the weight right

Frankly, losing weight successfully and staying in the BMI range of 20 to 25 is the most difficult instruction to follow for most diabetics. Most feel hungry all the time, and find it very hard to change the eating habits of a lifetime. But you must do it. Remember that those very habits have been largely what have brought on your diabetes in the first place. So do persevere. You can do it, and you are not on your own. Your dietician and family and friends will support you if you impress upon them how important it is for you.

How do you know if you are succeeding? Weigh yourself once a week, naked, on accurate bathroom scales, at the same time of day, under the same circumstances (say the same time after a meal). Measure round the widest part of your waist at the same time. Make a chart of both. And check your blood glucose level after different meals so that you learn which foods put it up more, and which ones less. If your attitude to these three simple actions is a good one, you will soon become enthusiastic about them and make progress. And as you do so, you will already be improving your blood glucose levels. After 2–3 months, you should even see your HbA1c (taken at your clinic visits) coming down.

Exercise

Eating correctly is only part of the weight loss programme. The other part is exercise.

As for type 1 diabetics, exercise is at least as important as the correct eating habits for type 2 diabetics – remember the hunter–gatherer theory? It is useful as a way of losing excess weight, but it is also especially useful as a direct aid to improving your sensitivity to insulin. The more exercise you do, the more efficient your muscles should become at taking up glucose and using it for energy, and the less you will need in the way of hypoglycaemic drugs or insulin. So just as becoming a normal weight is vital for you, so is the appropriate amount and type of exercise. You cannot afford to be a couch potato even if you are slim. You must exercise regularly, preferably on at least three or four days a week.

This does not mean slavishly adhering to some pre-arranged programme of exercising. It is a very rare person who can keep that up for long – and for you the change to regular exercise must be for life. So it must be the right exercise for you, in the right amount, and it must be safe.

In the past, doctors used to check the electrocardiograms of diabetics before advising them on the type of exercise they should do. That isn't considered quite so necessary as it was, as we have discovered that even people in heart failure can benefit from some exercise. But because type 2 diabetics, just like type 1 diabetics, are more prone than the general public to heart problems, to circulation problems in the eyes, kidneys and legs, and to difficulties with their peripheral nerves (neuropathy), it is advisable to choose your exercise carefully.

The first rule is that it isn't necessary for the exercise to be strenuous. Of course, if you like to run, that's fine, but a brisk walk is good for you and any increase from your previous physical activity will be of benefit. It is important for the exercise to be of the aerobic type, in which you are taking in plenty of oxygen while exercising against very little resistance. Walking, cycling, swimming, even ballroom dancing are good examples. Aerobics classes are fine if you make sure first that you can cope with their length and range of activity, so find out what you are letting yourself in for first. Avoid step aerobics as they put quite a lot of strain on the calf muscles and Achilles tendons: if you already have circulation problems an injury may make them worse.

A good start is to exercise (a walk, for example) for 30 minutes a day, then increase the time and pace as you feel fitter. Once it becomes a bit more strenuous, warm up and warm down appropriately, finishing with a good stretch. As with the weight and waistline, have an exercise chart, to keep you enthusiastic. And to prevent boredom, arrange to exercise with a friend, and vary it from time to time.

One important point about exercise – wear the best possible shoes for the job. That goes without saying for people without diabetes, but is particularly important for you, because you must keep your feet in good trim. The feet are often the weak spot in diabetes. The skin can so easily become infected, and they may be affected by poor circulation and by neuropathy, so that you don't notice when they are damaged. So take care of them – keep them clean and dry, with good nail care and free from athlete's foot, wear the proper socks (cotton, not nylon), and wear shoes that fit perfectly. Never compromise on shoes: they are the most important part of your clothing.

Alcohol and smoking

If you think I have been strict with you so far on your lifestyle, wait until you have read this section! On alcohol and particularly cigarettes, there should be no compromise. You must stick to moderate amounts of alcohol, if any at all. The advice is the same as for type 1 diabetics (see p. 43 for details): you must never drink on an empty stomach, you should stick to one or two standard drinks per day, and never binge.

As for smoking, you absolutely have to be a non-smoker, and avoid nicotine like the plague. If you can't do that, then there's little point in you reading on because any health advice you take will be nullified by your tobacco habit.

Why are doctors like myself so severe on tobacco? Because we are constantly having to deal with the human wreckage it causes, particularly when people have diabetes of either type. Asked to devise a drug that attacks all the weak spots in diabetes, a mad scientist would only have to point to tobacco and its inhalation through the lungs. So if you are still a smoker and have diabetes of either type, the next chapter is just for you. Non-smokers can miss it out!

12

Why you mustn't smoke

Smoking is a stupid, suicidal habit for anyone, no matter how healthy. It is even worse, if that is possible, for people with diabetes, because it multiplies all the extra risks they face of heart disease, strokes and kidney disease. So if you are a smoker, you must be a non-smoker before you put this book down.

Harms from smoking

How, exactly does smoking harm you? Tobacco smoke contains carbon monoxide and nicotine. The first poisons the red blood cells, so that they cannot pick up and distribute much-needed oxygen to the organs and tissues, including the heart muscle. Carbon monoxide-affected red cells (in the 20-a-day smoker, nearly 20 per cent of red cells are carrying carbon monoxide instead of oxygen) are also stiffer than normal, so that they can't bend and flex through the smallest blood vessels. The carbon monoxide gas also directly poisons the heart muscle, so that it cannot contract properly and efficiently, thereby delivering a 'double whammy' of damage to it that a diabetic heart, already working under the disadvantage of high blood glucose and probably high blood pressure, can ill afford.

Nicotine causes small arteries to narrow, so that the blood flow through them slows. It raises blood glucose levels and blood cholesterol levels, thickening the blood and promoting the degenerative process in the artery walls that is already faster than normal in diabetes. Both nicotine and carbon monoxide encourage the blood to clot, multiplying the risks of coronary thrombosis and a thrombotic stroke even more.

Add to all this the tars that smoke deposits in the lungs, which further reduce the ability of red cells to pick up oxygen, and the scars and damage to the lungs that always in the end produce chronic bronchitis and sometimes induce cancer, and you have a formula for disaster.

Some facts and figures

Here are the bald facts about smoking. If they do not convince you to stop, then you may as well give up reading this book, because there is no point in being 'health conscious' if you continue to indulge in tobacco. Its ill effects will counterbalance any good that your doctors can do for you.

- Smoking causes more deaths from heart attacks than from lung cancer and bronchitis.
- People who smoke have two or three times the risk of a fatal heart attack than non-smokers. The risk rises with rising numbers of cigarettes smoked, and it is doubled if you are also a diabetic.
- Men under 45 who smoke 25 or more cigarettes a day have a ten to 15 times greater chance of death from an eventual heart attack than non-smoking men of the same age.
- About 40 per cent of all heavy smokers, even if they do not have diabetes, die before they reach 65. Of those who reach that age, many are disabled by bronchitis, angina, heart failure and leg amputations, all because they smoked. Diabetes makes all these risks from smoking much greater. Only 10 per cent of smokers survive in reasonable health to the age of 75. Most non-smokers reach 75 in good health.
- In Britain, 40 per cent of all cancer deaths are from lung cancer, which is very rare in non-smokers. In a study of more than 10,000 British male doctors, of the 441 who died from lung cancer only seven had never smoked. Only one non-smoker in 60 develops lung cancer: the figure for heavy smokers is one in six!
- Other cancers that are more common in smokers than in non-smokers include cancer of the tongue, the throat, the larynx, the pancreas, the kidney, the bladder and the cervix.

Excuses for not stopping

The very fact that you are reading this book means that you are taking an intelligent interest in your health. So after reading so far, it should be common sense to you not to smoke. Yet it is very difficult to stop, and many people who need an excuse for not stopping put up spurious arguments for their stance. Table 12.1 lists excuses that every doctor is tired of hearing, and my replies.

Table 12.1 Excuses for not stopping

Excuse for not stopping smoking	Rebuttal
My father (or my grandfather) smoked 20 a day and lived till he was 75.	Everyone knows someone like that, but they conveniently forget the many others they have known who died long before their time. The chances are that you will be one of them, rather than one of the lucky few.
People who don't smoke also have heart attacks.	True. There are other causes of heart attacks, but 70 per cent of all people under 65 admitted to coronary care with heart attacks are smokers, as are 91 per cent of people with angina considered for coronary bypass surgery.
I believe in moderation in all things, and I only smoke moderately.	That's rubbish. We don't accept moderation in mugging, or dangerous driving, or exposure to asbestos (which incidentally causes far fewer deaths from lung cancer than smoking). Younger men who are only moderate smokers are at a much higher risk of an immediate heart attack than non-smoking men of the same age. Women with diabetes are at a higher risk of heart attack than non-diabetic men of the same age.
I can cut down on cigarettes, but I can't stop.	It won't do you much good if you do. People who cut down usually inhale more from each cigarette and leave a smaller butt, so that they end up with the same blood levels of nicotine and carbon monoxide. You must stop completely.
I'm just as likely to be run over in the road as to die from my smoking.	In the UK about 15 people die on the roads each day. This contrasts with 100 deaths a day from lung cancer, 100 from chronic bronchitis and 100 from heart attacks, almost all of which are due to smoking. Of every 1,000 young men who smoke, on average one will be murdered, six will die on the roads, and 250 will die from their smoking habit. Increase those risks for men and women with diabetes.
I have to die from something.	In my experience this is always said by someone in good health. They no longer say it after their heart attack or stroke, or after they have coughed up blood.

Table 12.1 Continued

Excuse for not stopping smoking	Rebuttal
I don't want to be old, anyway.	We define 'old' differently as we grow older. Most of us would like to live a long time, without the inconvenience of being old. If we take care of ourselves on the way to becoming old we have at least laid the foundations for enjoying our old age.
I'd rather die of a heart attack than something else.	Most of us would like a fast, sudden death, but many heart attack victims leave a grieving partner in their early 50s to face 30 years of loneliness. Is that really what you wish?
Stress, not smoking, is the main cause of heart attacks.	Not true. Stress is very difficult to measure and it is very difficult to relate it to heart attack rates. In any case, you have to cope with stress, whether you smoke or not. Smoking is an extra burden that can never help, and it does not relieve stress. It isn't burning the candle at both ends that causes harm but burning the cigarette at one end.
I'll stop when I start to feel ill.	That would be fine if the first sign of illness were not a full blown heart attack from which more than a third die in the first four hours. It's too late to stop then.
I'll put on weight if I stop smoking.	You probably will, because your appetite will return and you will be able to taste food again. But if you have read the section in this book about changing your eating habits to control your diabetes better, than you will lose any extra weight anyway. In any case the benefits of stopping smoking far outweigh the few extra pounds you may put on.
I enjoy smoking and don't want to give it up.	Is that really true? Is that not just an excuse because you can't stop? Ask yourself what your real pleasure is in smoking, and try to be honest with the answer.
Cigarettes settle my nerves. If I stopped I'd have to take a tranquillizer.	Smoking is a prop, like a baby's dummy, but it solves nothing. It doesn't remove any causes of stress, and only makes things worse because it adds a promoter of bad health. And when you start to have symptoms, like the regular morning cough, it only makes you worry more. It will also make it more difficult for you to control your diabetes.

Table 12.1 Continued

Excuse for not stopping smoking	Rebuttal
I'll change to a pipe or cigar – they are safer.	Lifelong pipe and cigar smokers are less prone than cigarette smokers to heart attacks, but have five times the risk of lung cancer and ten times the risk of chronic bronchitis than non-smokers. Again, double these figures for diabetics. Cigarette smokers who switch to pipes or cigars continue to be at high risk of heart attack, probably because they inhale.
I've been smoking now for 30 years – it's too late to stop now.	It's not too late whenever you stop. The risk of sudden death from a first heart attack falls away very quickly after stopping, even after a lifetime of smoking. If you stop after surviving a heart attack then you halve the risk of a second heart attack. It takes longer to reduce your risk of lung cancer, but it falls by 80 per cent over the next 15 years, no matter how long you have been a smoker.
I wish I could stop. I've tried everything, but nothing has worked.	Stopping smoking isn't easy unless you really want to do it. You have to make the effort yourself, rather than think that someone else can do it for you. So you must be motivated. If the next few pages do not motivate you, then nothing will.

Stopping smoking

You must find the right reason to stop for yourself. For someone with diabetes it should surely include that your diabetes will be under much better control, and you will be giving yourself a much better chance of remaining healthy for much longer. But there are plenty of other reasons.

For teenagers, who see middle age and sickness as remote possibilities, and who see smoking as exciting and dangerous, the best attacks on smoking are the way it makes them look and smell. You can also add the environmental pollution of cigarette ends and the way big business exploits developing nations, keeping their populations in poverty while the business makes huge profits by putting land that should be growing food under tobacco cultivation. Pakistan uses 50,000 hectares (120,000 acres) and Brazil 200,000 hectares (500,000 acres) of their richest agricultural land to grow tobacco. And as the multinationals are now promoting their product very heavily to the developing world, no teenager who smokes can claim to be really concerned about the health of the developing world. This is often as persuasive an argument in convincing a teenager to stop smoking (or not to start) as any about health or looks.

For some older women, the key may be looks. Smoking ages people prematurely, causing wrinkles and giving a pale, pasty complexion. Women smokers experience the menopause at an earlier age, even in the mid-30s, which can destroy the plans of businesswomen to have their families after a time for their career.

For men and other women the prime motivation is better health. The statistics for non-diabetic men and women in their 60s who smoke are frightening enough, without bringing in diabetes to further worsen them. More than a third of smoking men fail to reach pension age – add many more to that figure if they also have diabetes of either type.

How to stop smoking

Let us assume you are now fully motivated. How do you stop? It is easy. You become a non-smoker, as if you have never smoked. You throw away all your cigarettes, and decide never to buy or accept another one. Announce the fact to all your friends, who will usually support you, and that's that. Most people find that they don't have true withdrawal symptoms, provided they are happy to stop. A few become agitated, irritable, nervous and can't sleep at night. But people who have had to stop for medical reasons, say, because they have been admitted to coronary care, hardly ever have withdrawal symptoms.

That strongly suggests that the withdrawal symptoms are psychological rather than physical. And if you are stopping because you have found you have diabetes, that is not too different from the coronary care scenario. If you can last a week or two without a smoke, you will probably never light up again. The desire to smoke will disappear as the levels of carbon monoxide, nicotine and tarry chemicals in your lungs, blood, brain and other organs gradually subside.

If you must stop gradually, plan ahead. Write down a diary of the cigarettes you will have, leaving out one or two each succeeding day, and stick to it. Carry nicotine chewing gum or get a patch if you must, but remember that the nicotine is still harmful. Don't look on gums and patches as a long-term alternative to a smoke. If you are having real difficulty stopping, ask your doctor for a prescription of bupropion (Zyban). You may be offered a two-month course of the drug. It can help, but is by no means infallible.

If you do use aids to stop (others include acupuncture and hypnosis), remember that they have no magical properties. They are a crutch to lean on while you make the determined effort to stop altogether. They cannot help if your will to stop is weak.

Recognize, too, that stopping smoking is not an end in itself. It is only part of your new way of life, which includes your new way of eating and exercise, and your new attitude to your future health. And you owe it not only to yourself but also to your partner, family and friends, because it will help to give them a healthier you for, we hope, years to come. You are not on your own. More than a million Britons have stopped smoking each year for the past 15 years. Only one adult in four now smokes (and fewer than one doctor in 20). By stopping you are joining the sensible majority.

13

Keeping glucose levels down in type 2 diabetes

Managing your diabetes of either type has two main aims. One is to avoid and ease the symptoms of your diabetes, and the other is to prevent its long-term complications. We have established that the first is best achieved, if possible, by keeping blood glucose levels as near to normal as possible, and that the main way to do that is by eating healthily, taking plenty of exercise, losing any excess weight, drinking only moderately and not smoking at all.

Unfortunately, this ideal advice doesn't always work. If you have type 2 diabetes you may find that, despite eating and exercising correctly and losing all your excess weight, your fasting blood glucose levels are still too high, and you still feel under par. Or you can't manage to get your weight down enough, because you find it difficult to obey your new rules on eating or exercise. Either way, your new lifestyle has not brought your blood glucose levels into good enough control. Your doctor will then consider prescribing drugs that will help.

Oral hypoglycaemic agents

Such drugs are called oral hypoglycaemic agents. They are swallowed as pills or capsules, and are *not* an alternative to, or a substitute for, a better lifestyle. You must continue to eat healthily, exercise regularly and lose any excess weight while you are taking them. Occasionally they are prescribed soon after diagnosis of type 2 diabetes, but only in cases thought to be relatively severe, with blood glucose levels above 17mmol/l. As a routine they are started when healthy eating, exercise and loss of weight have failed to bring glucose levels under control.

Hypoglycaemic agents are in four main groups – sulphonylureas, biguanides, the alpha-glucosidase inhibitor acarbose, and the glitazones. In general, sulphonylureas are used in people of normal weight or who have been obese and have lost enough weight to show that they are conforming reasonably well to new lifestyle advice. Metformin, the single biguanide that is left on the market (others were abandoned because of side effects), is the drug of choice in people that have been unable to lose enough weight, and who remain at least 20 per cent over their ideal weight (corresponding to a BMI of 30 or more).

Hypoglycaemic agents do bring down fasting and random glucose levels, but you must always continue to make regular checks on your blood glucose, and if you are taking metformin, you also need regular checks on your kidney function. Oral hypoglycaemic agents are *not* useful, and are indeed never prescribed, in type 1 diabetes, and if they do not control type 2 diabetes satisfactorily, despite increasing doses, changing the drug or combining them with other hypoglycaemic agents, then they should be stopped. Insulin is then used instead. There is no reason to use two different sulphonylureas together, but either metformin or the alpha-glucosidase inhibitor acarbose may be added to a sulphonylurea if it has not adequately controlled the diabetes.

Sulphonylureas

Sulphonylureas probably act by inducing the pancreas to release more insulin, though in long-term treatment they may also reduce insulin resistance. The current sulphonylureas include glibenclamide (Daonil, Euglucon), gliclazide (Diamicron), glimepiride (Amaryl), and glipizide (Minodiab, Glibeneze). They differ from each other in their potency and length of action, so that they vary in strength of dose and in the numbers of times per day they should be taken. For example, glimepiride needs to be taken only once a day, while the others are usually given twice daily. Your diabetes specialist will assess for you the one that suits you best, and may change the prescription after an initial assessment period, depending on the success of the results and how you feel on the drug.

All sulphonylureas can cause hypo attacks, so you should be aware of the possibility and know about your particular early warning symptoms, such as sweating, shaking, palpitations, hunger and perhaps pins and needles around the mouth. This is particularly true for older people, who may have very little in the way of hypo symptoms. Because of this, some diabetic specialists prefer not to prescribe sulphonylureas in the elderly.

If you are starting to have a hypo, immediately swallow the equivalent of 15g of glucose. That is approximately a glass of lemonade or fruit juice, three heaped teaspoons of sugar, two barley sugars or five jelly beans. This can be repeated in five minutes if there is no obvious effect, and followed by a meal of starch (pasta, brown rice, wholegrain bread) to prevent a repeat attack. The sulphonylurea dose should be reduced and the treatment reviewed.

Some people mistake anxiety attacks for hypos – the symptoms may be superficially similar. A blood glucose test done during the attack should correct this mistake.

More serious than a mistaken anxiety attack is a hypo that comes on without any warning. This is labelled medically as hypoglycaemia unawareness or asymptomatic hypoglycaemia. It can happen to anyone treated with insulin or sulphonylureas, and the symptoms are the sudden onset of very peculiar behaviour or sudden loss of consciousness. The diagnosis is made from the low blood glucose reading taken with the patient's own kit, so it is advisable for people who are prone to such sudden hypos always to carry upon them their kit and instructions on what to do if found in such a state.

The treatment for hypoglycaemia unawareness is crucial. Do not try to pour liquid glucose into the mouth, as it may be inhaled and choke the patient. A smear of glucose gel, or failing that, honey, on the gums may help. The best treatment is an intravenous injection of dextrose, followed if necessary by a glucose drip. An alternative is an injection of a standard dose of glucagon deep into a muscle. Doctors carry glucose and glucagon in their emergency bags. A case could be made for the close relatives of someone with frequent hypos like this to learn how to inject glucagon themselves. However, adjustment of the sulphonylurea dose to avoid future attacks is better still.

An increased appetite and the tendency to hypoglycaemia on sulphonylureas give some people a tendency to weight gain: they should be on guard against this becoming excessive. If you reach good blood glucose control on a sulphonylurea, then you should consider reducing the dose or doing without it altogether, particularly if you are overweight. Sulphonylurea side effects are few, the commonest being mild indigestion or gastric upsets.

It used to be recommended that sulphonylureas be given 30 minutes before meals. Now it is accepted that they can be taken during meals. They may interfere with the action of the anticoagulant drug warfarin (a treatment to prevent thromboses after heart attacks, strokes and heart surgery) so sulphonylureas and warfarin are not usually given together – people taking warfarin are usually prescribed metformin or acarbose (or both) instead.

Biguanides

The biguanide metformin (Glucophage) delays the absorption of glucose from the gut into the bloodstream, interferes with the production of glucose from glycogen and fat stores in the liver, and increases the uptake of glucose from the bloodstream into the tissues. It therefore has three beneficial actions in type 2 diabetes. It is usually given as the drug of first choice for type 2 diabetes in people who remain 20 per cent or more overweight. It can also be given with a sulphonylurea or with acarbose, because the different effects of the three types of drug are complementary.

Metformin is given twice a day, usually starting at a dose of 500mg. The maximum dose is 1g twice daily. Its common side effects include loss of appetite, nausea and diarrhoea, which occur in around one in twelve patients (8 per cent). However, the mild loss of appetite may even be useful in most patients, considering that they are usually overweight in the first place. Less common is a metallic taste in the mouth, and an anaemia related to its interference with vitamin B12 absorption. An advantage of metformin is that its reduction of blood glucose levels is never enough to cause a hypo attack when prescribed on its own. It should be given with or after meals to avoid stomach upsets.

A very rare side effect of metformin is lactic acidosis. This is a life-threatening emergency, in which the patient becomes suddenly very ill. However, it is virtually confined to the very old, to people with kidney or liver disease and to people who are in heart failure or have severe peripheral vascular disease (such as pre-gangrenous changes in the feet). So people who are at risk of lactic acidosis from metformin are usually on a close watch for the early signs of the condition. Lactic acidosis was the reason for the withdrawal of a previous biguanide, phenformin, from the market: it was shown at the time that metformin was much less likely to cause it.

Acarbose

Acarbose (Glucobay), an alpha-glucosidase inhibitor, is one of a kind. It acts by delaying the conversion of sugars into glucose in the gut, so that the rise in blood glucose after a meal is much slower than usual and reaches a lower peak. Because of this action, acarbose also reduces the amount of insulin produced by the pancreas in response to a meal, so that it not only reduces blood glucose levels, it also reduces the high blood insulin levels in people with early type 2 diabetes. Trials have shown that acarbose also reduces HbA1c levels to a moderate degree (say from 9 per cent down to 8 per cent). It is given either alone or along with a sulphonylurea or metformin.

By starting it at a low dose that is gradually increased, the main side effects of acarbose, diarrhoea and wind, can be kept to a minimum. They usually subside if the treatment is continued, especially if you avoid eating foods containing simple sugars like glucose and sucrose.

Most people start on 50mg three times a day, then gradually increase it to 100mg or, less often, 200mg.

Rosiglitazone

Rosiglitazone (Avandia) was introduced in the UK in 2000 as a development of the sulphonylureas. Classified as a thiazolidinedione, it reduces blood glucose levels by reducing insulin resistance in fatty tissues, muscles and the liver. In theory, therefore, it is correcting the defect specific to type 2 diabetes. So far it only has a licence for use as a second agent to be given along with metformin in obese patients for whom metformin alone has not produced satisfactory diabetes control, or with a sulphonylurea in patients who cannot tolerate metformin or who cannot have metformin for other reasons (such as warfarin therapy).

It can be taken once or twice daily, with or without food. Its main problem is that it can cause fluid retention, which can induce heart failure, or make it worse, in susceptible patients. Patients also need to be monitored regularly for liver problems, since there have been a very few reports that it may cause jaundice. This can be avoided if blood tests are taken for liver enzymes, a rise in which is an early sign of a liver reaction. If the drug is stopped at this point, the reaction will reverse and no harm will be done. The advantage of adding rosiglitazone to either a sulphonylurea or metformin is much better blood glucose control. However, its effect on heart failure has led the UK authorities to warn doctors against giving rosiglitazone to patients with heart failure, or even with a past history of heart failure, and to patients with coronary symptoms or known coronary heart disease. The warning was extended in 2008 to patients with peripheral vascular disease (difficulties in the circulation of the arms and legs). As many people with diabetes also have incipient heart and circulation problems, these warnings have greatly reduced the drug's use.

Newer antidiabetic drugs

Rosiglitazone was followed by pioglitazone (Actos, Competact), which has all the restrictions set for rosiglitazone. Sitagliptin (Januvia) and vildagliptin (Galvus, Eucreas) are newer drugs unrelated chemically to the other antidiabetics; they are licensed to be given as an addition to metformin when it has not been able to control the diabetes adequately. They are said to increase insulin secretion. They carry similar warnings to those for rosiglitazone and pioglitazone, including the rare adverse effect of liver toxicity.

Exenatide (Byetta) is an injection that helps type 2 diabetes by increasing insulin secretion and slowing the emptying of the stomach, thereby tending to 'flatten' the rise of blood glucose after meals. It is recommended only as an addition to other treatments when good glucose control has not been achieved.

The time for insulin

If, despite the change in your eating habits, the extra exercise, the loss of weight and the various uses of sulphonylureas, metformin, acarbose and rosiglitazone, or the newer drugs, you still can't get your blood glucose under control, you may have to start on insulin injections.

Your doctor will first of all try to find out why the attempts at good control have failed. The commonest cause is failure to stick to the correct eating pattern. If that is due to ignorance of what you should be eating or of why you should be doing it, then reading this book should have helped. Failure to take the tablets regularly is the second commonest cause of poor diabetes control. Do try to follow the instructions. Go to the extent of having a small alarm on your watch if necessary, to remind you of the pill-taking time each day.

Emotional stress is yet another cause of poor control. It may cause you to revert back to your old lifestyle – eating badly, drinking more, going back to cigarettes. Or the extra adrenaline and anxiety may have a direct effect on your glucose levels. So recognize the times when you may need to monitor your glucose levels more closely, and act upon them. And get advice about how to manage your stress from the appropriate person in your professional diabetes team.

Illnesses such as infections (like severe influenza, gastroenteritis or a urinary infection) and an overactive thyroid (thyrotoxicosis) may cause you to lose your blood glucose control. If so, the correct action is to get help urgently: this is no time to increase doses of, or change, your hypoglycaemic agent. It is much safer to go on insulin for a while until the illness is brought under control. Your diabetes team will give you very detailed advice on how to do that.

There are a few people with newly diagnosed type 2 diabetes whose blood glucose fails to respond to any of the oral hypoglycaemic agents. This is called primary failure of oral treatment: such people need to be put on insulin permanently. Insulin may be needed, too, in the very small number of type 2 diabetics who lose their control for no obvious reason after having managed it well for years with hypoglycaemic agents. This is secondary failure. Many patients with primary or secondary failure actually may have an unusual form of type 1 diabetes that develops slowly after an onset that seems like the type 2 disease.

If you have type 2 diabetes that has begun to need insulin, and causes like infection, thyroid disease or severe stress have been ruled out, then you should consider yourself as a type 1 patient and organize your life accordingly. The first half of this book explains how to do it.

Most people who have to go on to insulin after oral treatment manage well on a single dose of longer-acting insulin per day, and can combine it with a hypoglycaemic agent. The transition period on to insulin is usually managed with the patient being a day patient at the diabetes centre or clinic, or even by visits to the home, each morning until the control is adequate. As with type 1 diabetes, the insulin dose is adjusted according to the blood glucose levels. It is best to keep the insulin dose as low as possible, as higher doses (say more than 50 units per day) will raise blood insulin levels, which could make your metabolic syndrome worse by tending to raise blood pressure and worsening the blood cholesterol profile.

As the UKPDS study showed, it is vital to manage these other issues as well as possible, on top of getting the glucose control right. How that is done today is the subject of Chapter 14.

Good glucose control

You may be wondering, however, before you read on, what actually is 'good' and what is 'bad' glucose control. With type 2 diabetes, you should be doing pre- and post-meal blood glucose tests once or twice a week, even if you are well controlled. If the control is less than good, or you are changing your treatment, you need to test more often.

The ideal fasting and after-meal blood glucose levels are, respectively, under 6mmol/l and under 8mmol/l. These levels go with an HbA1c under 7 per cent and no glucose in the urine test. We accept as 'good' control pre-meal and post-meal blood glucose levels of, respectively, under 8mmol/l and under 11mmol/l and an HbA1c between 7 per cent and 7.9 per cent. Levels above these are considered to range from fair control to poor control (this last defined as pre-meal and post-meal blood glucose levels above, respectively, 10mmol/l and above 13mmol/l, with more than one plus of glucose in the urine and an HbA1c of more than 9 per cent).

If you are not in the good or ideal group, then you need to do much better, and to review all aspects of your lifestyle, weight and treatment.

If you leave yourself in the fair or poor control group, you face very high risks. There are always ways to improve, and you should be very serious in doing so.

14

Keeping the complications at bay

As mentioned at the beginning of Chapter 13, every diabetic, whether with type 1 or type 2, has two aims. The first, to keep blood glucose levels as near normal as possible, was dealt with in that chapter. The second, how to keep the complications of the disease at bay, is dealt with in this chapter. It applies as much to people with type 1 diabetes as to those with type 2 disease.

The UKPDS study described in Chapter 10 proved that keeping blood pressure down is vital to preventing the complications that plague people with both types of diabetes: heart attacks, strokes, kidney disease, blindness and peripheral vascular disease (which leads to amputations). There is plenty of other evidence from studies of the link between abnormal blood cholesterol levels, which affect many people with type 2 diabetes, and heart disease that correcting abnormal blood cholesterol levels is just as important.

Of course, eating healthily and exercising regularly can bring the blood pressure down and go a long way to correcting the cholesterol profile, but for many people they are not enough. Their blood pressure remains too high and their cholesterol levels remain wrong. They need help from antihypertensive (blood pressure-lowering) drugs and hypolipidaemic (cholesterol-lowering) drugs.

Antihypertensive drugs

Learning about antihypertensive drugs is as easy as A, B, C, D. A stands for ACE inhibitors, B for beta-blockers, C for calcium antagonists (also known as calcium channel blockers), and D for diuretics. They all lower blood pressure by different mechanisms, so that if one does not hit the target blood pressure for you, it can be combined with one or two of the others. Combinations of drugs almost always finally bring the blood pressure down into the area that gives the least risk of heart attack, stroke, kidney failure, blindness and amputation from peripheral circulation problems.

Until the UKPDS results, many experts in diabetes preferred to choose the ACE inhibitors and calcium antagonists over the beta-blockers and diuretics as their first choice because of fears that the beta-blockers and diuretics might make the metabolic syndrome worse (by worsening the glucose and lipid profiles). However, UKPDS compared the beta-blocker atenolol with the ACE inhibitor captopril, and the drugs were equally effective. The conclusion was that the important factor in reducing long-term risks was the lowering of the blood pressure itself, and not the type of drug that reduced it.

One rule about the choice of antihypertensive agent still stands, however. If there is any evidence of kidney disease (such as micro-albuminuria) an ACE inhibitor, which has properties that protect the kidney, is the drug of first choice.

The aim of all high blood pressure treatment is to bring it down into the normal range. For diabetes of either type that means a figure below 130/80mmHg if possible, and certainly below 140/90mmHg. A detailed explanation of how these figures are arrived at is outside the remit of this book, but if you wish to know more, please see *Living with High Blood Pressure* (published by Sheldon Press in 2001), in which the latest guidelines of the International Hypertension Society are reported.

Your diabetes team will favour for their patients a particular group of drugs and drug combinations in which they have special expertise, and they will choose the drug or drugs they consider to be suitable for you. What is important is not the drug you are taking, but how effective it is at bringing down, and keeping down, your blood pressure. If the first drugs do not achieve their target blood pressures, their doses may be raised or other drugs may be added. Your diabetes team will be following strict guidelines on when and how to raise the doses or add new drugs, so be patient. It may take several months to gain full control, but in the vast majority of patients it is achieved in the end.

When taking your antihypertensive tablets, please follow the instructions carefully. Keep in mind that your blood pressure control is just as important as your blood glucose control in helping you avoid heart attacks, strokes, blindness, kidney failure and amputations in the future. You cannot tell from how you feel whether your blood pressure is high or low. The only way to know is by measuring it, so that has to be done weekly for a while until it is stable, then at least monthly after that. Never miss your blood pressure appointment.

Controlling cholesterol

What is cholesterol?

How the lipids (fats) in the blood affect your risk of future heart attacks and strokes is a complex subject that needs another whole book for a detailed explanation. It is enough to say here that fats in the blood are carried around the body linked to proteins called lipoproteins. Cholesterol is a fat, so that it is transported as a cholesterol–lipoprotein. Cholesterol–lipoprotein combinations are classified according to their physical structure, which makes a difference to the density (basically the 'hardness' or 'softness') of the fatty globules that float in your bloodstream.

Types of cholesterol and measuring blood lipids

They therefore may be high-density lipoprotein (HDL) cholesterol or low-density lipoprotein (LDL) cholesterol; others included in routine laboratory analysis are very low-density lipoprotein (VLDL) cholesterol and intermediate density lipoprotein (IDL) cholesterol. Total cholesterol level is simply the sum of them all. Fat is also transported around the body, as triglycerides (TG).

Put simply (the story is a bit more complex than explained here, but this is a practical system that can be used to determine risk of heart disease), LDL cholesterol and TG are the 'bad' lipids, and HDL cholesterol is the 'good' lipid. LDL cholesterol and TG are involved in depositing fats into artery walls, while HDL cholesterol removes the fatty material from the arteries.

So a high LDL cholesterol and TG with a low HDL cholesterol is a bad pattern of lipids that increases your risk of heart attacks and strokes. Make the LDL cholesterol and TG lower and the HDL cholesterol higher and you reduce the risks of heart attack and stroke. This is precisely the aim of lipid-lowering drugs. Many trials in many thousands of people with and without diabetes have shown that lowering total cholesterol levels (most cholesterol is in the form of LDL cholesterol, so that generally lowering cholesterol will lower LDL cholesterol the most) cuts deaths from heart attacks and strokes by around 30–40 per cent.

So, when you have your blood cholesterol checked routinely the total cholesterol is often the figure used to see how much you are at risk. Any total cholesterol figure above 5.5mmol/l is considered high and needs treatment. The usual treatment is advice on lifestyle change (healthier eating and more exercise) and, if this does not succeed, cholesterol-lowering drugs are considered if the total cholesterol figure remains above 6mmol/l.

High cholesterol and diabetes

If you have diabetes, this relatively easy-going advice given to most non-diabetics is not nearly enough. If your lipid levels are high, you have a greater need to reduce them than non-diabetics, because your chances of having heart attacks and strokes are so much higher.

The standard target for people with diabetes is a total cholesterol below 5mmol/l and a TG level below 2mmol/l. TG is important, as it tends to be much higher than normal in type 2 diabetes, and is usually linked to low HDL cholesterol levels. The two measurements of high TG and low HDL cholesterol together add considerably to your risk of heart disease and stroke, and they can be present without the total cholesterol level being abnormally high.

So for people with diabetes, even though total cholesterol may not be raised, their TG and HDL cholesterol levels may be such that they need treatment. This is why many diabetes clinics now treat on the basis of a 'lipid profile' that measures all the different forms of cholesterol, including TG, and not just total cholesterol alone.

Of particular importance is that the lipid abnormalities (in TG and HDL cholesterol especially) in diabetes often appear long before the onset of symptoms has led to the diagnosis. Diabetics face two to four times the risk of coronary heart disease of non-diabetics, an excess related more to the lipid problem than to the high blood glucose or even the high blood pressure. Treating the lipid abnormalities in diabetes is therefore extremely important.

In type 2 diabetes, hypoglycaemic agents like sulphonylureas and metformin reduce TG levels a little, but have no significant effect on other lipids. They are not an option for those with type 1 diabetes. Increasing exercise and losing weight does lower TG and raise HDL cholesterol, but not necessarily to the required levels. Many people with diabetes need drugs to complete the job.

Lipid-lowering drugs

The choice of drugs to correct the lipids lies between statins and fibrates. They both lower LDL cholesterol and TG levels and raise HDL cholesterol levels. The current tendency is to use fibrates to lower excessively high TG and to use statins to lower LDL cholesterol. Some patients may need both, but it is rare to recommend that they be taken together.

The choice of drug depends largely on your lipid profile and on the experience of the diabetes team in handling the different drugs. As at 2009 there are five statins (atorvastatin, fluvastatin, pravastatin, rosuvastatin and simvastatin) and four fibrates (bezofibrate, ciprofibrate, fenofibrate and gemfibrozil) on the market. They differ in their details but only slightly in their effects on blood lipids. It is now clear not only that they change lipid profiles towards a pattern linked to far fewer heart attacks and strokes, but also that their use reduces the numbers of heart attacks and strokes by between a third and a half.

Triglyceride levels and alcohol

A last point about lipid levels. Some people have raised TG levels, but their HDL cholesterol and LDL cholesterol levels are in the normal range. This pattern is mostly caused by overindulgence in alcohol, so do not be surprised or annoyed if your doctor, faced with these results, suggests that you cut down severely on your drinking.

15

Complications of diabetes

Up to this point, the book has been all about how to prevent the complications of diabetes, but it has not spelled out in detail what the complications are. Throughout the book there has been a repeated theme. People with diabetes of either type hardly ever die nowadays from the immediate consequences of poor glucose control, but they do die early from strokes, heart attacks and kidney failure, and they go blind and have nerve problems and circulation problems needing, sometimes, amputations.

This chapter reviews how these complications happen, and how, when they do happen, they can be treated.

Microvascular complications

We split up the complications of diabetes into microvascular and macrovascular events. In microvascular complications, the smallest blood vessels in the body become thickened, narrowed and fragile, so that it is very easy for the blood to clot within them, blocking off the circulation beyond the clot, or for bleeds to occur from them, damaging the tissues immediately around the bleed.

Microvascular disease is especially damaging to two organs, the eyes and the kidneys. In the eyes this is called retinopathy and in the kidneys it is called nephropathy. It also affects the nerves to the limbs, so that the brain receives the wrong messages from the nerves. This is peripheral neuropathy.

Diabetic retinopathy

Diabetic retinopathy can be diagnosed and followed up by using an ophthalmoscope to look at the retina. Instead of the usual network of clearly defined blood vessels against a smooth pink background, the doctor can see small 'aneurysms' (like tiny red blebs) on or beside the blood vessels. There may be smudges of red that represent bleeds, and paler 'exudates', often like bits of cotton wool, which are areas of leakage of fluids into the tissues. Repeated eye examinations will show whether the condition is worsening, stable or even improving with treatment. If it does become much worse, extensive laying down of new blood vessels inside the eye and deterioration in the centre of the retina leads to blindness.

Early retinopathy is seen in a quarter of diabetics on the day they are diagnosed, so the process has started long before the diabetes itself is obvious. Within eight years of diagnosis, half of all diabetics show some retinopathy, and after 20 years, almost every diabetic shows some signs of it. This should not depress you. Nowadays very few type 1 or type 2 diabetics become blind, because those with early retinopathy are followed very closely, and impending trouble can usually be prevented by new techniques such as laser treatment to deal with those new blood vessels and bleeding points.

So if you have been told you have some signs of retinopathy, don't worry about it. But do be very strict about your eye tests. Everyone with diabetes must have an annual eye examination and go for more frequent tests if they find that their vision is worsening. If retinopathy is diagnosed, it is usual for them to have a test every 6 months or more frequently, depending on its severity and progression.

During the test for retinopathy, you will also be checked for early cataract development. Cataracts are also a common complication of diabetes of either type. New techniques to replace cataracts with artificial lenses are a vast improvement on the old and have greatly improved the outlook for people with diabetes who a generation ago would have been virtually blind.

It can't be stressed enough that if you have retinopathy you can do a lot for yourself by very close control of your blood glucose levels. The huge US Diabetes Control and Complication Trial (DCCT) proved beyond all doubt that good control delayed the start and slowed the progression of all three microvascular complications (retinopathy, nephropathy and neuropathy). Reducing HbA1c levels from 9 per cent to 7 per cent (proof of good control) reduced the risks of all three by a massive 60 per cent. So if you have been diagnosed as having any of these complications, you have an extra incentive to control your diabetes better.

Diabetic nephropathy

Like retinopathy, diabetic nephropathy starts to affect the kidney before the diabetes itself is recognized. For many years it causes no noticeable symptoms at all, but it is easily detectable because the microscopic changes in the affected kidneys cause them to 'leak' tiny amounts of protein into the urine. This is picked up on a routine urine test for microalbuminuria.

The detection of anything over 30mg of protein in a litre (30mg/l) of urine is defined as microalbuminuria. It means that you are at risk of future kidney disease, and also at particular risk of the macrovascular complications of heart attacks and strokes.

The natural history of microalbuminuria is for it to worsen over years. Eventually enough protein is leaked into the urine for it to be detected by a normal protein 'dipstick' test (which is at least a ten-fold increase on the microalbuminuria level). From that point it is about seven years to complete kidney failure, needing dialysis and transplant.

Happily this progression can be stopped with a combination of excellent control of blood glucose and blood pressure. The aim for everyone with microalbuminuria is to have a blood pressure around 120/80mmHg or even below. There is good evidence that this greatly improves the long-term for them, in particular helping to avoid eventual kidney failure. The blood pressure will probably fall somewhat with good glucose control and regular exercise, but many experts now recommend that ACE inhibitors be used, too, not just because they bring down the pressure further, but also because they seem specifically to protect the kidney against further deterioration.

Once you have been found to have microalbuminuria, you must have regular blood tests to check your kidney function for the rest of your life. They will show if and how fast your kidneys are deteriorating and will be a guide to how best to manage it. Never miss your kidney tests. They are vital to your future.

Diabetic neuropathy

Diabetic neuropathy usually takes the form of loss of the ability to sense pain and temperature in a 'stocking and glove' pattern, starting first in the feet then spreading to the hands. Other symptoms include numbness, a burning sensation and feelings of pins and needles, that start in the toes and fingers and spread into the hands and feet. The symptoms are often worst at night. Many people with diabetes have minor forms of neuropathy without knowing it, the problem only coming to light when a doctor tests for it.

The main problem for people with neuropathy is that because you can't feel things going wrong with a foot, for example, you may not take the usual precautions against small injuries, infections or burns. I've known a man who lost half of his foot when a coal from the fire fell upon it. He was only made aware of his injury when he smelled the burning flesh.

That was an extreme case. Much more common are neglected small sores that develop into ulcers, and athlete's foot that doesn't itch, and so spreads until it is almost impossible to get a cure.

Neuropathic ulcers are 'punched out' open wounds under the pressure pads below the foot, the heel, or on the 'knuckles' or tips of the toes. They need to be treated by specialists in foot care to clean them out, but also to treat any infection and to take off the pressure that caused the ulcer.

If you have neuropathy, you must take special care of your feet. You must keep them clean and dry, examine them for any sores, bruises or infection several times a week, and regularly see the chiropodist (podiatrist) associated with your diabetes team. If you have any physical problems, like poor eyesight or muscle weakness or shaking, don't cut your own toenails: you need the professional to do this.

It can't be repeated too often that the best way to control neuropathy, as with retinopathy and nephropathy, is to keep your blood glucose levels as close to normal as possible. It isn't easy to ease the nerve symptoms once they have started, but some people find that daily doses of tricyclic drugs (more commonly used to treat depression), the anti-epilepsy drugs carbamazepine (Tegretol) or phenytoin (Epanutin),or a specific anti-neuropathic drug, gabapentin, help to reduce pain and the pins and needles. They do not appear to improve the numbness, however, so they are no substitute for meticulous foot care.

Painful neuropathy that hasn't been helped by paracetamol or the drugs mentioned above can sometimes respond to capsaicin cream: it does feel as if the skin is burning, but many people prefer that to the neuropathic pain. The last resort for very painful neuropathic pain is the group of opioid drugs that includes oxycodone and tramadol, but it is easy to become habituated to them, so you should only take them strictly as your diabetes team suggests.

Macrovascular complications

All through the book I have been harping on about heart attacks and strokes. They are what doctors define as the macrovascular complications of diabetes. Why they should particularly affect people with either type of diabetes is now quite clear. The constant contact of the artery walls with too much glucose, too much of the wrong types of fat, excessively high blood pressure, and in smokers nicotine, carbon monoxide and chemicals from tars all combine to accelerate the process that happens to everyone through life – atherosclerosis.

Even in apparently normal non-diabetic people, the process of atherosclerosis starts early in life, building up irregular and rough deposits of cholesterol- and triglyceride-laden fats in the lining of arteries throughout the body. Post-mortem examinations of young American soldiers killed in the Korean war showed that they all had the beginnings of atherosclerosis, even as young as 18. There were streaks of fatty deposits in their coronary and brain arteries. As these streaks change and increase in size and number, they form the basis of 'plaques' – raised and roughened areas of weakness in the artery wall. Eventually, at one of these weak spots a clot forms to block the vessel, or the vessel wall splits, so that it bleeds into the surrounding tissues. If these incidents occur in the coronary artery they cause a heart attack. In the brain they cause a stroke.

Atherosclerosis is universal in modern humans, but it is accelerated in diabetes. Age for age, people with diabetes have more plaques than people without it, and the plaques affect more arteries and are at a more advanced stage. This not only explains why diabetics have more heart attacks and strokes than others, but also why they need amputations. The atheromatous process spreads into the arteries to the legs and feet, too, blocking off the circulation to them. This leads to poor circulation which, if not controlled and improved, ends as gangrene and the inevitability of amputation.

As we all get older our risks of having a heart attack or stroke increases, decade by decade, from the age of 40 onwards, but the upward slope of the increase is much steeper for diabetics than for non-diabetics.

For women with diabetes the story is even worse. In the non-diabetic population, atherosclerosis is less severe in women than in men of the same age. A rough approximation is that women have a ten-year advantage in the progression of their atherosclerosis over men, so that women of 60 have the same risk of heart attack and stroke as men of 50.

It is not so for women with diabetes. Their diabetes seems to cancel out their natural advantage over men, a protection thought to have been provided by their sex hormones throughout their middle years. In fact diabetic women in middle age are at higher risk of heart attacks and strokes than non-diabetic men of the same age.

We know very well the causes of the extra risks of heart attack and stroke. They are cigarette smoking, obesity, high blood pressure, high blood cholesterol levels, poor control of diabetes and lack of exercise with a sedentary lifestyle. Tackle all of these together in the way this book has described, and you will hugely reduce your risk of all the macrovascular complications of your diabetes.

Peripheral vascular disease: foot problems

An extra word is needed here on the peripheral circulation – the arteries to the feet. Whether or not you have neuropathy (see p. 107), if you have diabetes you are at high risk of having peripheral vascular disease (atherosclerosis of the arteries in the legs). This shows itself in pain in the legs on walking any distance, and in long-standing ulcers and infections that don't respond well or fast to the usual treatments. Foot problems due to peripheral vascular disease account for a quarter of the admissions to hospital of all people with diabetes.

Your doctor and diabetes nurse will know something about your circulation from feeling the pulses in your groin, behind the knees, at your ankles and on the top of your feet. They can confirm suspicions of peripheral vascular disease by ultrasound and X-ray tests (angiography) of the circulation in your legs. If you are found to have peripheral vascular disease, you absolutely *must* stop smoking and avoid other people's smoke. Smoking is the biggest factor in promoting peripheral vascular disease. If you continue with it, you will certainly lose your legs, and probably your life, as it strongly correlates with fatal heart attacks in amputees.

Diabetic peripheral vascular disease, unsurprisingly, is treated with good glucose control, lowering blood pressure, attending to cholesterol levels and, as far as possible, improving exercise levels. That may be difficult if you already have pain on walking, but it is best to try to improve your walking distance gradually with a planned exercise programme.

Aspirin

If you do have diabetes with early signs of macrovascular disease, whether it has produced angina (heart pain on exercise) or peripheral problems (pain in the calves while walking) it may be worthwhile taking an aspirin a day. Aspirin, by preventing blood clots and protecting artery walls, has a good track record in preventing repeated heart attacks in non-diabetics with proven coronary heart disease, and it is now recommended for all diabetics presumed to be at higher than usual risk of macrovascular disease. To be frank, this means most people with either type 1 or type 2 diabetes, so many family doctors now advise all their diabetics to take a single 75mg aspirin tablet each day. It is difficult to know for sure that this is an advantage for people with no obvious symptoms, but there is good evidence that anyone already with proven heart and other arterial disease should take it. It may also help to slow the progress of retinopathy and nephropathy. The only people with diabetes in our local clinics who do not take aspirin are those who can't tolerate it, usually because it irritates their stomach or because they have had a previous stomach bleed after taking it.

Less common problems

The commonest form of diabetic neuropathy is described above (see p. 107). Other neuropathies are less common, but they deserve mention.

Mononeuritis

One is mononeuritis, a condition affecting a single nerve. This can be the nerve to one of the eye muscles, so that you develop a squint. Or it may affect the nerve to the shoulder or the nerve to the buttocks and thighs, so that the muscles are first very painful, then become weak and waste away. This is called 'neuralgic amyotrophy'. It can leave the shoulder or the buttock and thigh weakened and even paralysed for several months, but it usually recovers, quite suddenly, up to 18 months or two years later.

Autonomic neuropathy

In autonomic neuropathy the nerves affected are those controlling regulation of blood pressure, digestion and bladder. People with autonomic neuropathy may faint when standing from a lying or sitting position because of a sudden drop in blood pressure (postural hypotension), or they may have bouts of diarrhoea or an inability to pass urine when they wish to. They may sweat profusely after meals. Autonomic neuropathy has no specific treatment except for better glucose control, so if you have it, you usually have to live with it. But if you ever have to have an operation you must tell the anaesthetist beforehand, since it can lead to complications with the anaesthetic.

Sexual problems

Probably the best known and most worrying of the neuropathies that affect diabetics is impotence (erectile dysfunction) in men and loss of previous enjoyment in love-making (not loss of libido, necessarily) in women. If this is one of your problems, please tell your diabetes team about it: most people keep it secret, and it is certainly treatable. The problem in both sexes seems to be a mixture of neuropathy and peripheral vascular disease affecting the nerves and circulation to the genital organs. Impotence is a very obvious failure in men. Only in the past few years, however, has it been understood that the clitoris is a much larger organ in women than was thought. Bigger even than the erect penis, it extends up into the vagina, and surrounds it in a tube of tissue that erects when filled with blood, just like the penis, when the woman is sexually excited.

The importance of this information (discovered by two female Australian anatomists in 2000) is that it explains why women, as well as men, with sexual problems due to neuropathy can derive great benefit from sildefanil (Viagra), the anti-impotence drug. In Britain, impotence associated with diabetes is an official indication for sildefanil. Many doctors are now finding it to be successful in women with the corresponding problem.

16

Diabetes in pregnancy

Anna, one of the people with diabetes described in Chapter 2, had gestational diabetes. This is not strictly true diabetes, because her only problem was the finding of glucose in her urine, and it did not lead to overt diabetes. However, she was advised to follow a strict healthy eating and exercise regimen, mainly to prevent any complications during the pregnancy. She was then followed up for a year or two, to ensure that true diabetes did not develop afterwards. Her diagnosis of gestational diabetes remains in her medical records for future reference, as 40 per cent of women with gestational diabetes later become diabetic.

However, what about the woman who already has diabetes and who has become pregnant? Many women with type 1 diabetes in particular face problems in pregnancy, including rapidly worsening kidney disease and eyesight.

They should therefore not undertake becoming pregnant lightly. They should weigh up the pros (usually the great desire to have a child) with the cons (substantial deterioration in their diabetes control and the possibility of permanent deterioration of their physical condition).

If you do become pregnant, see your doctor immediately, so that you and your diabetes team can plan ahead. Don't wait the usual eight weeks or so to sign up at the antenatal clinic. If you have type 2 diabetes, for example, you may well have to go on insulin, since oral drugs are not given during pregnancy. An after-meal blood glucose level persistently above 8mmol/l suggests you need to go on insulin.

You must expect at some time in the pregnancy for your diabetes control to go haywire, so expect to be admitted to hospital during the pregnancy to change your insulin dose or to deal with unexpected hyper or hypo attacks.

Don't, if you are pregnant, try to cope with all the problems yourself. You will have emergency phone numbers to ring, 24 hours a day, so use them if you have doubts. When the baby is born, he or she is likely to be bigger than normal, often over 4.5kg (10lb), and to be less active than babies born of non-diabetic mothers. This is usual, and not a sign that the baby will be diabetic, but the consequence of the extra glucose he has been exposed to in the womb. It does no long-term harm, and is usually coped with quite routinely by the staff caring for the newborn.

After the birth, you will be faced with how to feed the baby. Choose the breast, by all means, but discuss the difference that will make to your blood glucose control with your diabetes team, and change your routine accordingly. Remember that while looking after a small child you cannot afford to have hypos or hypers, so you have an extra responsibility to keep your diabetes under good control.

Useful people and organizations

If you have diabetes you must be in regular contact with your local diabetes team. It comprises a minimum of a general practitioner, a dietitian, a diabetes nurse, a podiatrist (the newer name for chiropodist) and an ophthalmologist, who are there for all the routine tasks described in the book, and a diabetes specialist for the times when extra help is needed.

Your team will be a great source of addresses of and contacts with local organizations that can help in providing support when it is needed. The most important national organization for British diabetics is Diabetes UK (formerly the British Diabetic Association), to which all diabetics and their families should belong. Diabetes UK combines funding research with educational programmes for everyone with diabetes and their families, and has contact with over 4000 local groups, who provide the personal touch. There must be one in your area.

Diabetes UK
Macleod House
10 Parkway
London NW1 7AA
Tel.: 020 7424 1000
Membership enquiries: 0845 123 2399 (9 a.m. to 5 p.m., Monday to Friday)
Careline: 0845 120 2960 (9 a.m. to 5 p.m., Monday to Friday, responding to members' personal questions and concerns)
Website: www.diabetes.org.uk

For just £10.50 a year, your membership offers a bi-monthly magazine (*Balance*), and other publications and booklets on management of diabetes. In addition, when you have a chronic illness such as diabetes it is often difficult to insure yourself; Diabetes UK specializes in obtaining insurance for its members.

Index